Black Women and Breast Cancer

Anthropology of Well-Being
Individual, Community, Society

Series Editor: Ben G. Blount

Mission Statement

Well-being is central and important in people's daily lives and life history. This book series brings about understanding of what the complex concepts of well-being include. The concepts of quality of life, life satisfaction, and happiness will be explored and viewed at the individual level, the community level, and the level of society. The series encourages and promotes research into the concept of well-being, how it appears to be defined culturally, and how it is utilized across levels and across different social, economic, and ethnic groups. Understandings of how well-being promotes stability and resilience will also be critical to advances in understanding, as well as how well-being can be implemented as a goal in resisting vulnerabilities and in adaptation. Series books include monographs and edited collections by a range of academics, from rising scholars to experts in relevant fields.

Titles in the Series

Intimate Partner Violence and Advocate Response: Redefining Love in Western Belize, by Melissa Beske
Contemporary Conversations on Immigration in the United States: The View from Prince George's County, Maryland, by Judith Noemí Freidenberg
Cultural Dimensions of Well-Being: Therapy Animals as Healers, by Clementine K. Fujimura and Simone Nommensen
Love in the Time of Ethnography, edited by Lucinda Carspecken
Black Women and Breast Cancer: A Cultural Theology, by Elizabeth Williams

Black Women and Breast Cancer

A Cultural Theology

Elizabeth A. Williams

LEXINGTON BOOKS
Lanham • Boulder • New York • London

Published by Lexington Books
An imprint of The Rowman & Littlefield Publishing Group, Inc.
4501 Forbes Boulevard, Suite 200, Lanham, Maryland 20706
www.rowman.com

6 Tinworth Street, London SE11 5AL, United Kingdom

British Library Cataloguing in Publication Information Available

Library of Congress Cataloging-in-Publication Data
Names: Williams, Elizabeth A., 1972– author.
Title: Black women and breast cancer : a cultural theology / Elizabeth A. Williams.
Description: Lanham : Lexington Books, [2019] | Series: Anthropology of well-being individual, community, society | Includes bibliographical references and index.
Identifiers: LCCN 2018049935 (print) | LCCN 2018052995 (ebook) | ISBN 9781498561075 (electronic) | ISBN 9781498561068 (cloth : alk. paper)
Subjects: LCSH: Breast—Cancer. | African American women—Medical care. | Breast—Cancer—Religious aspects. | Health education.
Classification: LCC RC280.B8 (ebook) | LCC RC280.B8 W463 2019 (print) | DDC 616.99/449—dc23
LC record available at https://lccn.loc.gov/2018049935

∞™ The paper used in this publication meets the minimum requirements of American National Standard for Information Sciences Permanence of Paper for Printed Library Materials, ANSI/NISO Z39.48-1992.

Printed in the United States of America

This book is dedicated to Maggie Blair, Zeporah Elizabeth Gilley Booker, Annie Lou Williams, Fannie L. Swan, Mary Kelton Smith, Dr. Krystal Fraizer, Robin Jackman-Jenkins, and all Black women whose faith in God and complex hope allows them to prevail.

Contents

Preface ix

Acknowledgments xiii

Introduction 1

I: The God of Black Women and Breast Cancer **17**

1 Talking God and Talking Cancer 19

2 The Power of Black Women's Cancer Testimonies 43

3 Black Women's Cancer Support Seeking 55

4 Healing Claims as Acts of Faith and Resistance 73

II: Black Women Respond to God and Breast Cancer **85**

5 Black Women Transformed into Cancer Survivors 87

6 Black Cancer Survivors' Transformative Theology of Hope 125

Conclusion 149

Bibliography 155

Index 163

About the Author 167

Preface

For more than fifteen years I have been closely embedded with a locally organized group of seventy African American breast cancer survivors as an applied medical anthropologist and academic researcher. I have for years attended their monthly support group meetings and participated in public events hosted by the group. When asked, I have facilitated workshops, served as mistress of ceremonies at group functions, referred and connected members to health-care resources, co-written grant proposals, developed inspirational materials with/for and co-presented with members at breast cancer-related affairs. Over the course of these years I have also worked with a core group of twenty survivors in conjunction with my own research, as well as in relation to community-based participatory research projects I have been involved with as part of a federally funded, multi-site academic cancer research partnership. These mutually supportive interactions have fostered relationships that are more than those of research participants and researcher. This group and its members see me in many ways as one of their own. I am their resident breast cancer survivor advocate; I do not take this role lightly.

In addition to this group, my ideas about Black women and breast cancer have been shaped by my regular engagement over this period with a surgeon and oncologist who specifically treat women's cancers. Through our shared work and commitments to Black women's health, often as part of workshops, panels, or radio discussions to increase awareness about women's cancers in African American communities, we have had lots of conversations about breast cancer disparities and African American women. We have, over the years, had lively conversations about what responsibilities as Black women researchers and health-care providers mean in supporting the health and healing of cancer survivors. A recurring theme in these conversations is that unless Black women advocate for their concerns to be heard and addressed in health-care delivery spaces and research by both health-care providers and researchers, their needs often will go unmet. Unless Black women speak for themselves, no one else is likely to speak up for them.

This orientation to speak up for the medically underserved has shaped my professional career as a cancer survivor advocate. For more than eight years I served as a senior public health official within a state public health department, developing and advocating for policies to address health inequities, including cancer health disparities. I crisscrossed the state listening to those touched by cancer disparities and learning how to transform these concerns into programs and prevention models to reduce disparities and improve health outcomes. This work and my commitment to lifting up the concerns of the marginalized led to my appointment in an academic cancer center as a senior-level administrator. In this role, I championed the needs of medically underserved populations in cancer care, research, prevention, and control. Serving as a cultural broker between underserved populations and this complex comprehensive cancer center, seen as a behemoth by many in these communities, I became the voice for those whose voice might otherwise not have been considered in cancer care.

Through my ties to medical, research, and underserved communities, I served as an advisor for several years on a multicultural advisory committee for a globally recognized breast cancer advocacy organization, one named for the founder's sister who succumbed to breast cancer. In this role, I advocated for Black women's breast cancer prevention and control, health-care, and survivorship needs, including direct, face-to-face lobbying in the halls of the U.S. Congress. This experience provided strategic opportunities for me to further advocate for Black women's breast cancer needs through service on scientific research panels and setting of the organization's research and funding priorities, along with establishing a priority for breast cancer research that serves Black women and medically underserved populations by creating research mechanisms on breast cancer disparities and training opportunities for underserved breast cancer–disparities investigators. In each of these, my focus was on creating spaces for the marginalized to be seen, heard, and supported. This is what I do. I do this because I believe that Black women have the right to flourish.

Immersion into the lives of Black women with breast cancer for me, not just as a researcher and administrator, has also occurred through regular attendance at Black church worship services. During Pink Sunday worship services, those usually held in October, and others in Black Protestant churches, I have invariably heard Black women give breast cancer testimonies. These testimonies often include a profession of their faith in God, specific examples of how God intervenes in their cancer experiences, and why being a living witness as a breast cancer survivor and sharing their public testimony is important. I have witnessed my fair share of clergy members' laying on hands and congregational prayers of healing, support, and deliverance after the newly diagnosed give their public testimonies. As further displays of solidarity and support, I have witnessed congregations, bedecked in pink, sing songs of deliverance, participate in litanies about healing, and listen to preachers give homilies about divine healing using biblical and extra-biblical texts for their exegeses. These services concretely make the personal the political when it comes to talking about breast cancer and Black communities. What I have discovered, being present in these contexts, is that when you pay attention to Black women with respect and interest, Black women often talk and open up their lives to you in important ways.

As a licensed clergy in the United Methodist Church for more than ten years, I have been with people at the most vulnerable times in their lives. This includes breast cancer survivors across the breast cancer spectrum from diagnosis through dying and death. Because I regularly encounter Black women who have been diagnosed with breast cancer who know me as clergy, I have in church and non-church settings been asked to pray with women experiencing breast cancer. Often these prayers are preceded or followed by Black women's telling me their stories. Because they believe I care, they talk. And in turn, I listen. What they say further extends my insight into the cultural theology of Black women and breast cancer. Their ideas about God and what God does for them are ideas I wrestle with in theology classes in divinity school. As an academically trained theologian, my interest in Black women's theology and its application to issues of health, healing, and wholeness is more than a hobby. It is part of my praxis as an anthropologically trained theologian and pastor. I think, work, and serve Black women who see and rely on God has a resource for life itself. Understanding and interpreting who God is, what God can do, and what difference this makes for Black women are bread and butter issues for the Christian church. These are the ties that bind me to this work of interpreting African American women's cultural theology of breast cancer.

Acknowledgments

This work would not have been possible without the support of the African American breast cancer survivors who shared their lives and stories with me over these many years. The best of whatever I am as an applied scholar and theologian is because of them. Thank you Sisters Network Nashville and the Cervical Cancer Coalition of Tennessee for allowing me to be co-laborer in supporting cancer survivors and achieving health equity for those touched by cancer.

I am also indebted to several institutions and colleagues for supporting my endeavors, including my forever mentors, Dr. John van Willigen, Dr. Fon Gordon, Hattie M. Scott, Robbie M. Jackman, and Rev. Dr. Warren G. Booker Jr.; Tennessee State University; Dr. Lesia Crumpton-Young and the 2017 and 2018 Tennessee State University Summer Faculty Writing Retreats; Tennessee State University Department of Public Health, Health Administration, and Health Sciences; Dr. Mohamed Kanu, Dr. Elizabeth Brown, Professor Wanda Burrell, Deborah McCauley, Dr. Revlon Briggs, Dr. Kimberlee Wyche-Etheridge, Dr. Theodora Pinnock, Sharon Kay, Xuam Lawson, Carlice Knox, John Ferguson, Katina Beard, Rev. Michelle Morton, Rev. Linnie Junita Booker, Rev. Dr. Herbert Lester, Rev. Anthony Henderson, Tonya Micah, Kenneth Sessions, Clark Memorial United Methodist Church, Beulah Baptist Church, and Vanderbilt University Divinity School. Thank you for always believing in me, most especially when I doubted myself.

Special thanks goes to Kasey Beduhn, Alison Keefner, and the entire Lexington Books team for their guidance throughout the editorial and publishing process. I am particularly grateful to an anonymous reader whose thoughtful comments and suggestions made this a richer text and affirmed the importance of this work.

I would like to express special thanks to my family: my parents and greatest cheerleaders, Drs. Charles and Hilda Williams; my brother, Charles Christopher Williams, and other brothers, Travis Garrett and Robert Watson, for always encouraging me; and to the wind beneath my wings, my niece and nephews, Arriana Danielle Williams, Brennon Christopher Williams, and Kylan Isaiah Warren for making my heart smile and giving me the courage to soar.

Introduction

Christian theology at its core is a story about someone being in trouble. In response to this trouble, God intervenes. God identifies with those in trouble, walking with them through the experience. Yet, the God of Christian theology goes a step further. God prevails over trouble. God is an overcomer. Black women with breast cancer identify with this God. They also see themselves in this theological narrative. They see themselves in the midst of troubles—troubles like racism, poverty, and environmental exposures that create the disease that affects their bodies. They see the troubles of breast cancer, their biological disposition toward more aggressive cancer types, later stage diagnoses, poorer cancer prognoses, diminished quality care, and worse outcomes.

Black women also palpably feel the troubles breast cancer brings—like fear, physical disfigurement, social isolation, being stereotyped for their treatment decisions, abandonment, and even death. Black women indeed feel the myriad troubles breast cancer brings. But, Black women also know God in their troubles. They know an active God who identifies with them, one who prioritizes them and their needs. They know this God, through scripture and experience, as a God who does not put them on the back burner, but instead puts them front and center. And because they know God as an overcomer and a creative force, they know themselves as overcomers. For with God, their troubles do not last always.

African American breast cancer survivors who subscribe to a belief in a triune God—one that includes God, as transcendent maker, creator, and sustainer; Jesus, as embodied redeemer and overcomer; and the Holy Spirit, as transformative presence and power—map God onto their lives and bodies. In turn, God becomes a powerful cultural symbol for them. Cultural symbols like God, informed by religion and theology, support breast cancer survivors' meaning making and serve several important cognitive functions. At least four functions are served by cultural symbols, including symbols such as these: (1) "explanations," which elucidate relationships between objects, people, and events; (2) "rudimentary theoretical propositions," which are truisms and proverbs, which provide clear and uncomplicated explanations about life events and experiences; (3) "explicit theories," relatively complex explanations about the relationships among and within individuals and institutions; and (4) "symbolic universes," those which explain key existential dilemmas (i.e., meaning of life) and/or explain complex ideas about existential issues like survival.[1] Black women think and talk about God as a cultural symbol in all of these ways in the context of their breast cancer experiences.

Beyond cultural symbol, God also represents for Black women their entire cultural epistemology of breast cancer. They understand breast cancer based on what they think and know about God. What they know is that Jesus was a historical figure. What they believe is Jesus is the Christ, God incarnate. In light of what the Jesus of their faith endured—his suffering, crucifixion, and resurrection—and their own experiences, Jesus means freedom from bondage. As the womanist theologian Grant puts it, "Jesus means freedom from the sociopsychological, psychocultural, economic and political oppression of Black people."[2] In this way God serves as a "global meaning,"[3] which provides stable beliefs and values that influence their explanations of events and understanding of experiences. For Black breast cancer survivors Jesus represents the totalizing experience of breast cancer—pain, disfigurement, death, dying, hope, triumph, and new life. Jesus is a sign of what they believe about life, death, disease and overcoming. The Holy Spirit also represents what these Black women think about their faith in God—faith about who they are in the present and hope about who they will be after breast cancer. For many Black women with breast cancer, God is a complex cultural symbol of knowing, power, and hope. In fact, for these women, God in totality is "all things."[4]

The triune God is more than a set of ideas or a disembodied symbol for Black women. I argue that for Black women with breast cancer, their identification with the triune God is embodied. The noted theologian James Cone was among the first to identify Jesus's embodiment as Black.[5] Jesus's embodied blackness is not based on an ideological distortion of Jesus's ethnicity, but instead on the soteriological meaning of Jesus's Jewish heritage, as part of a people who endured slavery and the Exodus and were saved by the Hebrew God from the repression of Pharaoh.[6] Jesus is further identified socially as Black because of the parallels between Jesus's living under a repressive government, unjust treatment and subjection to violence, and unjust crucifixion and the experiences of African Americans in the United States.[7] Thus Jesus's solidarity with the "least of the people" is affirmed in his experience of living life with an oppressed status.

The significance of Jesus Christ for Black women is further rooted in his humanity. Jesus's significance is threefold: "first he identifies with the 'little people,' Black women, where they are; secondly he affirms the basic humanity of these, 'the least'; an thirdly, he inspires active hope in the struggle for resurrected, liberated existence."[8] Jesus's life and ministry, crucifixion, and resurrection are significant because they make absolutes like life, death, pain and suffering, and the oppressions of racism, classism, and sexism Black women experience concrete. God through Jesus Christ becomes concrete for Black women as the one who faces the challenges life presents. This means that Christ (and the entire triune God), interpreted in the experiences of Black women with breast cancer "is a Black woman."[9] Black woman with breast cancer, like God, become powerful beings that step into trouble and face it head on. As God made flesh, Black women respond to breast cancer as sentient and incarnate beings. Black women take on God's attributes and mannerisms, essentially becoming God in flesh in key areas of their lives such as in making treatment decisions or determining how they will live as cancer survivors. Black women identify in an embodied way with the living God while facing breast cancer.

Extending their embodied identification with the triune God, like Jesus of the first century CE, Black women, because of their ethnicity, class, and gender, live with social marginalization and being politically discounted. Black women with breast cancer, as Jesus, face testing and endure isolation. They, as Jesus, suffer undeservedly life's affronts as marginalized people. As Jesus, Black women with breast cancer are at times misunderstood, abandoned, persecuted, and even betrayed by those closest to them. Black women with breast cancer, as Jesus, face their own mortality. Black women sacrifice their flesh as Jesus, with physical scars to prove what they have experienced. And like Jesus, Black women face death, rise up in response, and are made anew. Black women with breast cancer live out the Christ story from beginning to end and identify with Jesus as "the divine co-sufferer, the one who empowers them in situations of oppression."[10]

Life after breast cancer for most Black women, similar to life after Jesus's resurrection, is never the same. Black women embody Christ renewed as breast cancer survivors. Most operate in new ways and with sustained drive, energy, and focus they did not know before. They imagine themselves empowered by the Holy Spirit. In tangible ways, Black women with breast cancer do not just espouse their Christian theology. They embody their theology through their troubles, endurance, and overcoming. Black women's cultural theology one, which knows God as sign, symbol, and promise of God's liberating freedom made flesh in trouble and triumph, is a practical theology. It is a practical theology because it is not separate from, but central to Black women's everyday lives. What Black women believe about God shows up in how they talk about God, what they say about themselves, how they talk about breast cancer and their responses to the disease. Accessing such an enmeshed cultural theology, rooted in Black women's spirituality and faith, requires immersion into Black women's lives, particularly those who have experienced breast cancer.

For this examination of Black breast cancer survivors' cultural theology, I have drawn on my professional experiences as an applied anthropologist and public health researcher, policy maker, academically trained theologian, and pastor. I have also made use of my professional experiences as an advocate for the medically underserved and champion for health equity for/with/in the breast cancer community. All of these aforementioned experiences and the corresponding social networks formed from them foster my interest in a Black women and their cultural theology of breast cancer. My decades-long work with an organized African American breast cancer support group has also proven especially helpful in grounding this theological study.

From this organized support group, I recruited members and others from their social networks to participate in focus groups, photo voice groups, and individual interviews that span over fifteen years. In total, twenty African American women, ranging in age from thirty-five to seventy-four years, served as key informants for this work. The women who participated in this study all self identify as Christian and are members of Protestant denominations, including Baptist, United Methodist, African Methodist Episcopal, and nondenominational churches. One study participant is a practicing Buddhist who, because of her early upbringing in Christian churches, nevertheless asserts core Christian beliefs as part of her faith orientation. The participants in this study include those with college degrees and some collegiate training as well as those with only high school diplomas. Professionally, the women in this study include those who are retired domestic workers, administrators, call center representatives, nurses, and ministers. All of the participants were born and raised in the Southeast United States and continue to live in the South.

For this study, I used anthropological methods, including participant observation of African American breast cancer support group meetings, public breast cancer events, and religious services, as a primary means of accessing Black women's words and embodied ideas about theology and to observe how theology is embedded in Black women's lives and survivorship. I combined these methods with principally Black feminist/womanist anthropological and womanist theological approaches. A Black feminist/womanist anthropological approach purposefully centers the experiences of Black women as sites for examining cultural phenomena, asserting that Black women's simultaneous locations as Black and female offer a distinct lens to understand the human condition.[11] In a related fashion, a womanist theological approach includes examining how Black women use African American biblical hermeneutics, Biblical texts, and Christian theology by rereading them as transgressive and transformative vehicles, which speak to the intersectionality of Black women's lives. As I see it, Black women use elements of Black feminist/womanist anthropology and womanist theology as critical lenses for interrogating and disrupting systemic oppressions that they experience (i.e., patriarchy, racism). Black feminist/womanist anthropology and womanist theology, as part of an investigative approach, offer a totalizing a way of understanding Black women's social location, transcendent and practical experiences of God, as well as their relationships with others.

Several things result from employing womanist theology and womanist theory as frameworks for considering Black women's theology and experiences with breast cancer. Importantly, Black feminist/womanist perspectives locate Black women's experiences as central to social scientific inquiry. Rather than objects of research, Black women become agents in theorizing about their experiences. Womanist theology takes this a step further by affirming Black women in asserting their right to challenge leadership as an exclusively male domain. What also comes from this latter womanist theological approach of rereading Black women's lives and experiences into sacred texts and Christian theology are that they challenge adversity and reject the oppressive and limiting social conditions and social roles that have defined Black women. Finally, what also emerges from this transgressive rereading of Black women's experiences as central and sacred texts are that it creates opportunities for Black women's leadership and their moral authority to exercise influence over their personal circumstances and relational lives with others, as empowered breast cancer survivors, to serve as the nexus for theological and social scientific investigation.[12]

To situate Black women's cultural theology of breast cancer, I have used social science and public health literature to make claims about who Black woman with breast cancer are, how the circumstances of being Black and female puts their health at risk, and how faith in God serves them. The decidedly theological approach of this study, informed by the social sciences, considers three essential questions about Black women, God and breast cancer—namely, (1) what troubles does breast cancer inflict on Black women? (2) Where is God in response to the troubles Black women with breast cancer experience? And finally, (3) what is Black women's response to God and the troubles breast cancer brings?

BLACK WOMEN AND THE TROUBLES OF BREAST CANCER

Why the story of Black women, breast cancer, and their theology is such an important one rests in part on Black women's breast cancer statistics in the United States and the stories behind the numbers. The 2018 American Cancer Society review of trends in breast cancer incidence and mortality, which features data from the National Cancer Institute's Surveillance, Epidemiology and End Results (SEER) Program, the Centers for Disease Control and Prevention's National Program of Cancer Registries, and the North American Association of Central Cancer Registries, provides a starting point for understanding the disease.[13] While the age-adjusted breast cancer incidence rates were parallel for Black women and white American women in the United States between the years 2010 and 2014 (128.7 versus 125.5 per 100,000), between 2010 and 2014 the breast cancer mortality rate was 8 percent higher for Black than white American women (29.5 versus 20.8 per 100,000).[14]

Breast cancer incidence among Black women, similar to white American women, increased steadily since the 1980s, in large part due to increased detection rates as a result of mammography screening.[15] Although white women have comparatively higher breast cancer incidence than African American women, the incidence rate among white women has stabilized in recent years, yet continued to increase among Black women.[16] Although the breast cancer incidence rate among Black women has increased slowly at a rate of 0.5 percent per year (1985–2012), the incidence rates for the two groups converged for the first time in 2013 with rates of 122 per 100,000 for Black women and 124 per 100,000 for white women.[17] At the same time the breast cancer incidence rate for Black women has risen, the median age of diagnosis among Black women remains younger, at fifty-eight years for Black women compared to sixty-two years for white women.[18] Likewise, the incidence rate for younger women diagnosed with breast cancer, those under the age of forty-five years, is higher for Black women compared to white women.[19]

In contrast to the incidence trends, the morality rate from breast cancer is significantly higher among Black women as an ethnic group compared to white women.[20] From 1989 to 2012, breast cancer death rates decreased by 36 percent, which translates to 249,000 breast cancer deaths averted in the United States over this period. This decrease in death rates was evident in all racial/ethnic groups except American Indians / Alaska Natives. However, the mortality disparity between Black and white women nationwide has continued to widen; and, by 2012, death rates were 42 percent higher in Black women than in white women.[21] Although not well understood, the commonly cited risk factors for Black women's higher mortality rates include molecular differences in breast cancer tumor types, socioeconomic status and poverty, differences in access to health care, and cultural factors.[22] African American women have a poorer prognosis when diagnosed with breast cancer when compared to white women at similar ages and across all breast cancer stages.[23] One of the most significant factors accounting for the breast cancer disparities African American women experience is their higher risk for specific cancer types, like triple-negative breast cancer.

Triple-negative breast cancer (TNBC) refers to invasive tumors that are negative for estrogen (ER) as well as progesterone and ERBB2. While only 15 percent of breast cancers in the United States have the triple-negative phenotype, Black women have a twofold higher population-based TNBC incidence rate compared to white American women in all age categories.[24] Patients with TNBC are not candidates for endocrine therapy or treatment with targeted ERBB2 agents. As a consequence, adjuvant breast cancer systemic therapy, like Tamoxifen citrate, which is a widely used adjuvant endocrine therapy for breast cancer that has been available since the 1970s, is not a viable treatment option for Black women with TNBC. This has severely limited the therapeutic options available for African American women with TNBC.

Using SEER data, Akinyemiju and colleagues have demonstrated that African American women with TNBC have worse outcomes compared to African American women without TNBC, in part because fewer adjuvant therapies are available.[25] The steadily increasing breast cancer incidence rates among African American women and their higher risk for TNBC are two important reasons for Black women's poorer mortality outcomes when compared to white American women. But molecular differences are not the only factors that increase Black women's risk for poorer breast cancer outcomes. Socioeconomic status and poverty are also major contributors to disparities in breast cancer outcomes for Black women.

African Americans experience poverty rates that are twice as high as those for white Americans in the United States (25.8 percent versus 11.6 percent).[26] Although overall uninsured rates for Americans declined from 16 percent in 2010 to 11.5 percent in 2014, disparities in insurance rates persist for Blacks with 11.9 percent of African Americans being uninsured compared to 8.2 percent of white Americans in 2014.[27] Differences in breast cancer mortality outcomes for African Americans have long been associated with lack of medical coverage, treatment-seeking delays, access to health care barriers, and other factors directly and indirectly related to socioeconomic status (e.g., geographic barriers to care, comorbidities).[28] Due to the synergistic effects of poverty, social environment, and health, Freeman and Chu have proposed a framework based on the social determinants of health for examining cancer disparities across the spectrum from prevention to post-treatment, survival, and morality. This framework includes social determinants, including poverty and low socioeconomic factors, social injustice, and culture, which directly affect Black women's breast cancer outcomes.[29]

Poverty and low socioeconomic status are associated with lack of access to resources, information, and knowledge, along with poor living conditions; risk-promoting lifestyles, attitudes, and behaviors; and limited access to health care.[30] In addition to having lower insurance rates than their white American counterparts, African Americans are also more likely to have inadequate insurance coverage. Although African Americans have benefited from the Affordable Care Act and the expansion of access to health care, racial and ethnic disparities in health-care access, while diminishing, nevertheless remain.[31] Uninsured and underinsured women are less likely to have core biopsies, lumpectomies, adjuvant therapy, and hormonal treatment,[32] are more likely to receive late-stage diagnosis[33] and are less likely to survive breast cancer.[34] These forms of poverty put Black women at increased risk for dying at greater rates from breast cancer.

Poverty not only creates access to care barriers, it also affects the types health behaviors Black women engage in that increase their susceptibility to breast cancer. Poverty is associated with lifestyles and environmental factors that contribute to morbidity and mortality.[35] African Americans and other racial/ethnic minorities are more likely to be affected by structural racism that harms their health, including living in communities with high concentrations of dilapidated houses, greater exposure to pollutant and toxins, and having limited opportunities for high-quality education and decent employment.[36] Lack of physical activity,[37] smoking, poor nutrition, alcohol consumption, and obesity[38] are factors that tend to be more prevalent among the socioeconomically disadvantaged and are identified risk factors for cancer development.[39] Obesity alone has been linked to increased risk of developing breast cancer.[40] Black women because of poor diet and lack of physical activity are more susceptible to weight gain, which plays a role in the development of breast cancer and survival rate for Black women.[41]

Barriers related to culture have also been identified as factors that increase Black women's risk for poorer breast cancer outcomes. Spiritual beliefs and practices feature prominently for many African Americans in coping with illness, restoring health, and in their health decision-making.[42] Many African American women assert their belief in God alone to make life and death decisions, for divine intervention in health challenges, and for promoting curing.[43] While Black women's reliance on their faith as a source of strength is positive, solely divulging their breast cancer symptoms to God can be detrimental if it deters Black women from seeking appropriate medical treatment and care.[44] Added to this, Black women compared to white American women are more likely to hold more pessimistic and fatalistic views about breast cancer treatment and have less confidence in Western biomedicine.[45]

Persistent race-based disparities in breast cancer outcomes have been observed,[46] which has led to increased focus on the relationship between racial discrimination and breast cancer disparities. Evidence suggests that racial prejudice and discrimination experienced by African American women in health care contributes to Black-white disparities in breast cancer mortality, including differential referrals for mammography screening and unequal delivery of breast cancer care.[47] Relatively little empirical research has been conducted examining direct associations between social injustice and Black women's breast cancer outcomes.

A study conducted by Taylor and colleagues using prospective data from the Black Women's Health Study identified a positive association between perceived racial discrimination and breast cancer incidence.[48] Young Black women, notably those under fifty years of age, who reported higher levels of racial discrimination, including everyday racial microaggressions and major discriminatory practices in areas of employment, housing, and interactions with the police, were at greater risk of subsequently developing breast cancer. The authors posit that perceived experiences of racism serve as chronic stressors that alter Black women's immune functioning and/or endogenous hormone levels, which may, in turn, increase breast cancer risk.[49]

Black women's breast cancer outcomes are also affected by how their providers perceive them. Physicians perceive patients based on race and socioeconomic status and take these into consideration when assessing patients' abilities to understand medical information or comply with medical recommendations and treatment protocols.[50] As a consequence physicians' differing perceptions may result in differences in quality of care provided.[51] Physicians who negatively perceive their patients may translate into differential access to breast cancer treatment and patient satisfaction with care. A study by Bickell and colleagues indicated that breast cancer patients who reported higher perceived racism during their interactions with health-care providers tended to also report lower satisfaction with their breast cancer care.[52]

African American women's experiences of racism, sexism, and classism extend beyond those experienced in health-care settings. Discrimination in the social environment further puts Black women's health at risk. Black women are historically a socially marginalized group in the United States who, as a consequence of their intersectional identities of race, class, and gender, are subject to disempowerment and violence.[53] One way Black women are socially disenfranchised is through what the Black feminist Patricia Hill Collins calls "controlling images" or social constructions of Black womanhood and femininity.[54] These controlling images reduce Black women's complexity to a set of racially gendered roles, responsibilities and expectations. A controlling image that affects Black women and their health is the "Strong Black Woman" image.[55] According to this schema, Black women are expected to be stoic, fearless, undeterred, and emotionally resolute in the face of adversity or everyday challenges. Undergirded by their faith in God, Black women who conform to this schema are perceived as unaffected by traumas or emotional upheavals.

The "Strong Black Woman" schema, while serving as a source of strength for Black women, can also be problematic for Black women who subscribe to or are expected to adhere to these roles by their families, peers, and community. Black women locked into this schema are less likely to reach out to others for support or to be emotionally vulnerable. This in turn increases their risk for greater psychological distress, depressive symptoms, obesity and cardiovascular risk.[56] Black women with breast cancer may be further at risk for these negative mental and physical health outcomes because of the ways breast cancer culture, spirituality, and Strong Black Woman ideas reinforce the concealment of their true feelings out of fear that they may be found to be socially unacceptable.[57]

In short, for all of these reasons and others, breast cancer is trouble for Black women because it reflects how the racial, political, economic, and social vulnerabilities Black women face increase their susceptibility to the disease and affects the breast cancer types they are more often diagnosed with. Breast cancer is also trouble for Black women because too often they receive poorer quality care and die at higher disease rates. Breast cancer is also trouble for Black women because it forces them to remain silent about what hurts them, disproportionately costing too many of them their health and lives. Breast cancer is too often a menace for Black women.

Yet, into the swirling mass of troubles that compromise Black women's health and well being, many could give up and succumb to the disease, but they don't. Why not? They don't give up because they see God in the trouble. They envision God using breast cancer to teach, guide, clarify, and heal them in their trouble. Where is God? God is in the struggle with them. And because God is in the struggle, Black women respond to God. Many respond by becoming God in flesh, distinctly identifying with the triune God. Instead of being defeated by breast cancer, many Black women are empowered to use their lives to challenge breast cancer, to speak up, to support others, and to trouble the troubles that cancer brings.

BLACK WOMEN'S SPIRITUALITY AND RELIGIOSITY

Black women's reliance on God as a resource for strength, clarity, and resolve in dealing with breast cancer is part of a larger tradition of spirituality and religiosity exercised among African Americans. African American spirituality and religiosity have historically been resources peoples of African descent in the United States use to survive the institution of American slavery, segregation, and overt, covert, and systemic forms of discrimination they faced.[58] As defined by Newlin, Knafl, and Melkus,

> [African American spirituality refers to] faith in an omnipotent, transcendent force; experienced internally and/or externally as caring interconnectedness with others, God, or a higher power; manifested as empowering transformation of and liberating consolation for life's adversities; and thereby inspiring fortified belief in and reliance on the benevolent source of unlimited potential.[59]

Similar, yet distinct from spirituality, *religiosity*, according to Mattis is defined as the "degree to which individuals adhere to the prescribed beliefs and practices of an organized religion."[60] Black women use both their spiritualty and religiosity in response to adversities, including health challenges like breast cancer. In fact, Mattis suggests that African American women in particular have a stronger focus on spirituality in their lives than African American men. This greater focus has been posited by Tate to be the consequence of the sexual abuse and frequent separation from family members African American women endured during slavery.[61] As a consequence, Black women came to revere God as both a healer and comforter in times of struggle.[62]

Throughout their experiences in the nineteenth and twentieth centuries, African American women have used formal religious involvement and private devotional practices (e.g., prayer, reading the Bible, listening to religious songs) to negotiate the range of human experiences and adversities they experienced, including racist, sexist, and classist oppressions,[63] illness, health decision-making,[64] psychosocial distress, and other life challenges.[65] Even for Black women who may not have been actively involved in organized religious life, prayer has served as a primary coping strategy in times of hardship.[66]

African American women have principally used spirituality and religiosity to cultivate hope in times of despair and adversity. For Black women, adversities often highlight tensions between reality and desire, the way things actually are and the way they hope for things to be. Yet what spirituality in combination with religiosity offers is a transcendent counterweight that permits Black women to generate alternative conceptualizations of life's possibilities. As Mattis in her qualitative study of African American women's meaning making and coping in response to adversity points out, spirituality "disrupts the semantic relationship between fact and truth."[67]

Through spirituality and religiosity, Black women with breast cancer distinguish between the social realities of their lives, including the impacts of the breast cancer (i.e., "fact") and what is possible for them by believing in God, namely surviving breast cancer (i.e., "truth"). While Black women with breast cancer are fully aware of the limitations they face (even their own mortality), those limitations do not bind them. Through their faith in God, Black women transcend their life circumstances by using their relationship with God as a means of (re)appraising their thoughts and experiences and to (re)envision and (re)create their destinies, including their lives during and beyond breast cancer.

This text considers the challenges Black women face, including those presented by breast cancer. These are challenges Black women turn to spirituality and religiosity in nuanced ways to extricate themselves from. Calling on God as a source and resource to make "a way out of no way," Black women construct their cultural theology by talking about God, not as academic theologians, but as women who experience God in the day-to-day practical and material realities of their lives.

The book, in the pages that follow, is divided into two thematic sections in line with the questions it seeks to answer. Part 1: The God of Black Women and Breast Cancer examines the troubles that Black women with breast cancer face and where they see a transcendent and practical God in those experiences. Black women's "God talking" and what semantic symbols of God Black women use are considered in chapter 1. Black women's cancer testimonies as lived texts out of which they build their cultural theology of God and breast cancer are explored in chapter 2. The racially gendered challenges African American women face in seeking psychosocial support for breast cancer and the role spirituality and religiosity play in overcoming these concerns are examined in chapter 3. Fatalism and how Black women think about healing as resistive responses are themes that focus chapter 4.

Part 2: Black Women Respond to God and Breast Cancer examines how Black women use an embodied theology and spirituality in response to breast cancer. Examining women's use of their cultural theology to envision different life possibilities, chapter 5 considers women's leadership, biblically centered women's advocacy roles, womanist ethics and the moral anthropology they offer Black women in asserting their authority to (re)actualize their lives as breast cancer survivors. The constellation of Black women's ideas about God, breast cancer, and themselves as God made flesh are brought together in chapter 6 into a systematic theology of complex hope—a simultaneously transcendent and materially grounded hope that Black breast cancer survivors create that emboldens them to persist in troubling the troubles that breast cancer brings.

NOTES

1. Berger, P., and Luckman, T. *The Social Construction of Reality.* Garden City, NY: Anchor, 1966.
2. Grant, J. (1989). "Experience Revisited: The Challenge of the Darker Sister." In *White Women's Christ and Black Women's Jesus: Feminist Christology and Womanist Response*, 195–230. Atlanta: Scholars Press.
3. Park, C., and Folkman, S. (1997). "Meaning in the Context of Stress and Coping." *Review of General Psychology*, *1*, 115–144.
4. Carter, H. (1976). *The Prayer Tradition of Black People.* Valley Forge, PA: Judson Press.
5. Cone, J. (2003). *God of the Oppressed.* Maryknoll, NY: Orbis Books.
6. Ibid.
7. Cone, J. (2011). *The Cross and the Lynching Tree.* Maryknoll, NY: Orbis Books.
8. Grant, "Experience Revisited," 217.
9. Ibid., 220.
10. Ibid., 212.

11. McClaurin, I. (Ed.). (2002). *Black Feminist Anthropology*. New Brunswick, NJ: Rutgers University Press.

12. Mattis, J. (2002). "Religion and Spirituality in the Meaning-Making and Coping Experiences of African American Women: A Qualitative Analysis." *Psychology of Women Quarterly*, *26*, 309–321.

13. Siegel, R., Miller, K., and Jemal, A. (2018). "Cancer Statistics, 2018." *CA: A Cancer Journal for Clinicians*, *68*, 7–30.

14. American Cancer Society. (2017). *Breast Cancer Facts & Figures 2017–2018*. Atlanta: American Cancer Society.

15. American Cancer Society. (2016). *Cancer Facts & Figures for African Americans, 2016–2018*. Atlanta: American Cancer Society.

16. Howlader, N., et al. "SEER Cancer Statistics Review, 1975–2012." November 2014. http://sser.cancer.gov/csr/1975_2012/ (accessed July 3, 2017).

17. DeSantis, C., Fedewa, S., Goding Sauer, A., Kramer, J., Smith, R., and Jamal, A. (2015). "Breast Cancer Statistics, 2015: Convergence of Incidence Rates Between Black and White Women." *CA: A Cancer Journal for Clinicians*, *66* (1): 31–42.

18. Ibid.

19. Newman, L., and Kaljee, L. (2017). "Health Disparities and Triple-Negative Breast Cancer in African American Women: A Review." *JAMA Surgery*, 485–493.

20. Yedjou, C., et al. (2017). "Assessing the Racial and Ethnic Disparities in Breast Cancer Mortality in the United States." *International Journal of Environmental Research and Public Health*, *14* (486): 1–14.

21. DeSantis, Fedewa, Goding Sauer, Kramer, Smith, and Jamal, A. "Breast Cancer Statistics, 2015."

22. Admuyiwa, F., Groman, A., O'Connor, T., Ambrosone, C., Watroba, N., and Edge, S. B. (2011). "Impact of Body Mass Index on Clinical Outcomes in Triple Negative Breast Cancer." *Cancer*, 4132–4140.

23. American Cancer Society. *Cancer Facts & Figures for African Americans, 2016–2018*.

24. Kohler, B., et al. (2015). "Annual Report to the Nation on the Status of Cancer, 1975–2011, Featuring Incidence of Breast Cancer Subtypes by Race/Ethnicity, Poverty, and State." *Journal of the National Cancer Institute*, *107* (6): djv048; and Amirikia, K., Mills, P., Bush, J., and Newman, L. (2011). "Higher Population-Based Incidence Rates of Triple-Negative Breast Cancer among Young African American Women: Implications for Breast Cancer Screening Recommendations." *Cancer*, *17* (12): 2747–2753.

25. Akinyemiju, T., Moore, J., and Altekruse, S. (2015). "Breast Cancer Survival in African-American Women by Hormone Receptor Subtypes." *Breast Cancer Research and Treatment*, *153* (1): 211–218.

26. Maccartney, S., Bishaw, A., and Fontenot, K. (2003, February). "Poverty Rates for Selected Detailed Race and Hispanic Groups by State and Place: 2007–2011; American Community Survey Briefs." Retrieved May 21, 2018, from American Community Series Brief/ 11–17: http://www.census.gov/prod/2013pubs/acsbr11-17.pdf.

27. Ward, B., Clarke, T., Freeman, G., and Schiller, J. (2015, June). "Early Release of Selected Estimates Based on Data from the 2014 National Health Interview Survey." Retrieved May 21, 2018, from Centers for Disease Control and Prevention: https://www.cdc.gov/nchs/data/nhis/earlyrelease/earlyrelease201506.pdf.

28. Yedjou, C., et al. "Assessing the Racial and Ethnic Disparities in Breast Cancer Mortality in the United States."

29. Ibid.; and Freeman, H., and Chu, K. (2005). "Determinants of Cancer Disparities: Barriers to Cancer Screening, Diagnosis, and Treatment." Surgical Oncology Clinics of North America , *14*, 655–669.

30. Gerend, M., and Pai, M. (2008). "Social Determinants of Black-White Disparities in Breast Cancer Mortality: A Review." *Cancer Epidemiology, Biomarkers & Prevention*, *17* (11): 2913–2923.

31. Chen, J., Vargas-Bustamante, A., Mortensen, K., and Ortega, A. (2016). "Racial and Ethnic Disparities in Health Care Access and Utilization under the Affordable Care Act." *Medical Care*, *54* (2): 140–146.

32. Su, S., et al. (2017). Quality of Invasive Breast Cancer Care for Low Reimbursement Rate Patients: A Retrospective Study." *PLoS ONE, 12* (9): 1–13.

33. Lukavsky, R., and Sariego, J. (2015). "Insurance Status Effects on Stage of Diagnosis and Surgical Options Used in the Treatment of Breast Cancer." *Southern Medical Journal, 108* (5): 258–261.

34. Zhang, Y., Franzini, L., Chan, W., Xu, H., and Du, X. (2015). "Effects on Health Insurance on Tumor Stage, Treatment, and Survival in Large Cohorts of Patients with Breast and Colorectal Cancer." *Journal of Health Care for the Poor and Underserved, 26* (4): 1336–1358.

35. Gerend and Pai. "Social Determinants of Black-White Disparities in Breast Cancer Mortality."

36. ·Bailey, Z., Krieger, N., Agenor, M., Graves, J., Linos, N., and Bassett, M. T. (2017). "Structural Racism and Health Inequities in the USA: Evidence and Interventions." *Lancet, 389*, 1453–1463.

37. Hair, B., Hays, S., Tse, C., Olshan, A., and Bell, M. (2014). "Racial Differences in Physical Activity among Breast Cancer Surviors: Implications for Breast Cancer Care." *Cancer, 120*, 2174–2182.

38. Thompson, C., Owusu, C., Nock, N., Li, L., and Berger, N. (2014). "Race, Age, and Obesity Disparities in Adult Physical Activity Levels in Breast Cancer Patients and Controls." *Frontiers in Public Health, 2*, 150.

39. Irigaray, P., et al. (2007). "Lifestyle-Related Factors and Environmental Agents Causing Cancer: An Overview." *Biomedicine & Pharmacotherapy, 61*, 640–658.

40. Ligibel, J. (2011). "Obesity and Breast Cancer." *Oncology, 25*, 994–1000.

41. Stolley, M., Sharp, L., Wells, A., Simon, N., and Schiffer, L. (2006). "Health Behaviors and Breast Cancer: Experiences of Urban African American Women." *Health Education & Behavior, 33*, 604–624.

42. Johnson, K., Elbert-Avila, K., and Tulsky, J. (2005). "The Influence of Spiritual Beliefs and Practices on the Treatment Preferences of African Americans: A Review of the Literature." *Journal of the American Geriatrics Society, 53*, 711–719.

43. Gerend and Pai. "Social Determinants of Black-White Disparities in Breast Cancer Mortality."

44. Gullatte, M., Brawley, O., Kinney, A., Powe, B., and Monney, K. (2010). "Religiosity, Spirituality, and Cancer Fatalism Beliefs on Delay in Breast Cancer Diagnosis in African American Women." *Journal of Religion and Health, 49* (1): 62–72.

45. Lannin, D., Mathews, H., Mitchel, J., and Swanson, M. (2002). "Impacting Cultural Attitudes in African-American Women to Decrease Breast Cancer Mortality." *American Journal of Surgery, 184*, 418–423.

46. DeSantis, Fedewa, Goding Sauer, Kramer, Smith, and Jamal. "Breast Cancer Statistics, 2015."

47. Freeman and Chu. "Determinants of Cancer Disparities."

48. Taylor, T., Williams, C., and Makambi, K. (2007). "Racial Discrimination and Breast Cancer Incidence in US Black Women: The Black Women's Health Study." *American Journal of Epidemiology, 166*, 46–54.

49. Gerend and Pai. "Social Determinants of Black-White Disparities in Breast Cancer Mortality."

50. Hall, W., et al. (2015). "Implicit Racial/Ethnic Bias among Health Care Professioals and Its Influence on Health Care Outcomes: A Systematic Review." *American Journal of Public Health, 105* (12): e60–76.

51. Ibid.; and Institute of Medicine. (2003). *Unequal Treatment: Confronting Racial and Ethnic Disparities in Health Care.* (B. Smedly, A. Stith, and A. Nelson, Eds.) Washington, DC: National Academies Press.

52. Bickell, N., Neuman, J., Fei, K., Franco, R., and Joseph, K. (2012). "Quality of Breast Cancer Care: Perception Versus Practice." *Journal of Clinical Oncology, 30* (5): 1791–1795.

53. Collins, P. H. (2000). *Black Feminist Thought.* New York: New York University Press; and White, E. (1990). *The Black Women's Health Book: Speaking for Ourselves.* Seattle: Seal Press.

54. Collins, *Black Feminist Thought.*

55. Abrams, J., Maxwell, M., Pope, M., and Belgrave, F. (2014). "Carrying the World with the Grace of a Lady and the Grit of a Warrior: Deepening Our Understanding of the 'Strong Black Woman' Schema." *Psychology of Women Quarterly, 38* (4): 503–518.

56. Ibid.; and Beauboefu-Lafontant, T. (2008). "Listening Past the Lies that Make Us Sick: A Voice-Centered Analysis of Strength and Depression and Black Women." *Qualitative Sociology*, 391–406.

57. Gatison, A. (2015). "The Pink and Black Experience: Lies that Make Us Suffer in Silence and Cost Us Our Lives." *Women's Studies in Communication, 38*, 135–140.

58. Lewis, L. (2008). "Spiritual Assessment in African-Americans: A Review of Measures of Spirituality Used in Health Research." *Journal of Religion & Health, 47*, 458–475.

59. Newlin, K., Knafl, M., and Melkus, G. (2002). "African-American Spirituality: A Concept Analysis." *Advances in Nursing Science, 25* (2): 57–70.

60. Mattis, J. (2000). "African American Women's Definitions of Spirituality and Religiosity." *Journal of Black Psychology, 26*, 101–122.

61. Tate, J. (2011). "The Role of Spiritualty in the Breast Cancer Experiences of African American Women." *Journal of Holistic Nursing, 29* (4): 249–255.

62. Musgrave, C., Allen, C., and Allen, G. (2002). "Spirituality and Health for Women of Color." *American Journal of Public Health, 92*, 557–560.

63. Higginbotham, E. (1997). "The Black Church: A Gender Perspective." In T. Fulop and A. Raboteau (Eds.), *African American Religion: Interpretive Essays in History and Culture*, 201–225. New York: Routledge; and McKay, N. (1989). "Nineteenth-Century Black Women's Spiritual Autobiographies: Religious Faith and Self-Empowerment." In Personal Narrative Group (Ed.), *Interpreting Women's Lives: Feminist Theory and Personal Narrative,* 139–154. Bloomington: Indiana University Press.

64. Hamilton, J., Galbraith, K., Best, N., Worthy, V., and Moore, A. (2015). "African-American Cancer Survivors' Use of Religious Beliefs to Positively Influence Utilization of Cancer Care." *Journal of Religion & Health, 54*, 1856–1869.

65. Hamilton, J., Moore, A., Johnson, K., and Koening, H. (2013). "Reading the Bible for Guidance, Comfort, and Strength during Stressful Life Events." *Nursing Research, 62* (3): 178–184; and Hamilton, J., Sandelowski, M., Moore, A., Agarwal, M., and Koenng, H. (2013). "'You Need a Song to Bring You Through': The Use of Religious Songs to Manage Stressful Life Events." *Gerontologist, 53* (1): 26–38.

66. Johnson, Elbert-Avila, and Tulsky."The Influence of Spiritual Beliefs and Practices on the Treatment Preferences of African Americans."

67. Mattis. "Religion and Spirituality in the Meaning-Making and Coping Experiences of African American Women," 314.

1

The God of Black Women and Breast Cancer

Chapter One

Talking God and Talking Cancer

Breast cancer for Black women brings a variety of experiences, both good and bad. In responding to both, Black women turn to theology, what they know and believe about God to make sense of it all. What African American women with breast cancer believe about God is often expressed in how they talk about God and breast cancer. When African American breast cancer survivors talk about God they are engaged in far more than idle conversation. What these cancer survivors are doing is constructive theology.

Not simply a vocation for academically trained theologians, constructive theology is fundamentally about articulating who God is, how God operates, who people are in relationship to God and each other (i.e., theological anthropology), and what this means for how people live. As such, constructive theology is a way of examining peoples' thoughts about God and the behavior that results from these thoughts. Examining beliefs and practices in this way is an inquisitive process, one where asking questions about God and seeking answers for application to human experience are important goals. Because the primary intent of constructive theology is application or what do we do because of what we believe, inquiry for constructive theology first presupposes that theological norms exist. Many Black breast cancer survivors talk about God because they believe in God, particularly the God that Christianity espouses.

Christian theology of the kind Black women with breast cancer talk about is part of a bounded and internally logical cultural system.[1] It is what Park and Folkman call a "global meaning," in that the God of Christian theology provides a totalizing way of making sense of human experience and guiding human action.[2] As a result, inquiries about Christian theology seek to understand the locus of belief, a belief system's contours, how the system shapes ways of knowing or epistemologies, and how to evaluate its faithfulness with human belief and agency. Several tools can be used to assess continuities and discontinuities between Christian beliefs and practices. These include scripture, tradition, reason, and experience. Which inquiry tool is used and how it is applied depends on the locations (i.e., social, historical, political) where "God talkers" are at work.[3] African American breast cancer survivors are indeed "God talkers" when it comes breast cancer. Talking about who God is and how God operates in human experience supports these survivors' well-being by providing an overarching framework for explaining how life works and how to respond to what happens in life.

Given that theological inquiry seeks to understand what affects people and what they do, it needs a template by which to guide its work. African American breast cancer survivors use scripture, experience, tradition, and reason together to guide their theological inquiries and locate God in the experience of cancer. Using the systematic theologian Peters's criteria for doctrinal faithfulness, scripture serves as a principal guide for Black women's theological inquiry.[4] Although scripture is itself a cultural construction, African American breast cancer survivors use their reading of scripture as the essential tool for testing the validity/faithfulness of their Christian beliefs and practices. Their reading of scripture often involves, in light of a womanist theology, locating themselves in these texts.

Scripture provides a basic framework and language for African American breast cancer survivors' theological work. Survivors regularly use scripture to articulate what they believe. They also use scripture to evaluate the faithfulness of what they do in relation to their reading of scripture and what scripture reveals to them. Black women breast cancer survivors in turn use scripture to guide the actions they take and the choices they make for their well-being.

Experience, as another theological tool, offers additional material for understanding the layered meaning(s) of scripture and Christian faith traditions Black women draw upon to sustain them. Black women use lived experience to evaluate scripture's relevancy. Experience is where scripture is put into action.

Tradition is the sum total of African American breast cancer survivors' beliefs and practices that manifest over time from individual and collective experiences. Tradition, as an additional theological tool, represents the beliefs shared by Christians, the Black faith tradition, and the broader community of African American breast cancer survivors about God and cancer. When Black women with breast cancer talk about God, what it evidences is that Black women have been talking about God and talking about breast cancer for a long time.

Lastly, reason is a final theological tool by which Black women question, understand, wrestle with and reconcile scripture and tradition in light of human experience. African American breast cancer survivors have lots of questions about God and cancer. In thinking carefully about cancer and through what they understand as divine revelation from God, Black women have also found some answers about God, breast cancer, and the way life works. So as a consequence they keep talking—about God and about breast cancer.

TALKING GOD: THE DUAL NATURE OF GOD AS "LIBERATOR" AND "JUDGE"

Talking about God is not easy. As a consequence theologians often use metaphors as stand-ins and approximations for God. African American breast cancer survivors, as theologians, do the same thing. They talk about God metaphorically. God as metaphor is an idea also reinforced in many African American churches where cancer survivors attend. God is often referred to as a "shepherd," a "doctor," or "provider." God takes on the nature and characteristics most closely related to the metaphor used. Different metaphors for God are evoked in response to specific contextual needs. Talking about God by using metaphors reflects, for many African American breast cancer survivors, God's omnipresence and God's nature as sovereign and omniscient.

When African American breast cancer survivors talk about God they use two primary metaphors, God as judge and God as liberator. The constructive theologian Brown-Douglass describes these metaphors.[5] Constructions of God as "judge" and "liberator" are well entrenched in African American Christian beliefs and African American theology.[6] As evidenced in African American constructive theology, particularly developed by womanist theologians, God as judge and liberator undergirds a broader set of cultural beliefs located within an African American "spirituality of survival."[7] In this spirituality of survival, God's natures as judge and liberator are inextricably tied to the day-to-day experiences of African American people.[8] As judge and liberator, God helps Black people make sense of what is going on and helps them cope with life's challenges. God's presence and ability to make a way out of no way for African American breast cancer survivors are essential to well-being.

The God as judge metaphor describes one type of dynamic relationship between God and African American breast cancer survivors important to well-being. As judge, God calls survivors to think about their behavior, especially behaviors considered antithetical to Christian ideals of moral correctness (i.e., hatred, bigotry, etc.). For these cancer survivors, God as judge acts not out of hatred. God is not vengeful or seeking retribution. Instead, God as judge gets people's attention out of love. Love accepts people as they are while also challenging people to be better. African American breast cancer survivors believe God desires the best for their well-being and challenges them to live in ways that support their well-being.

As a metaphorical liberator, God functions in other ways to precipitate Black breast cancer survivors' well-being. In this role, God frees people from oppressions (e.g., cancer). God does this for some African American breast cancer survivors by miraculously healing them from cancer. God liberates other survivors by helping them to persist through circumstances (i.e., undergoing cancer treatment). The nature of God as a metaphorical liberator is complex. As a liberator, God acts out of a sincere and heartfelt love for people. God's desire, as understood as part of African American constructive theology, is for people to be "whole."

In order to ensure wholeness happens, God delivers believers from circumstances and situations harmful to well-being. African American cancer survivors are not merely passive though. They are also active participants in reshaping their lives to achieve well-being. Cancer survivors become part of a way of living God outlines, which help them achieve and maintain wholeness as well as spiritual, physical, and emotional well-being. For African American breast cancer survivors who think this way, their health locus of control shifts fluidly between a survivor-centered (internal) and God-centered (external) view of their disease/illness.

In this theological study, Black cancer survivors did not always explicitly identify God by the metaphors of "judge" or "liberator." However, in talking about God's presence in their cancer experiences, they often evoked images, qualities, and behaviors that could very easily be used to characterize what judges or liberators do. Using a womanist theological approach, God as judge and God as liberator serve for the researcher as metaphorical devices for expressing a symbiotic relationship between God and African American breast cancer survivors. God talks and acts in these survivors' lives. Survivors in turn talk and act based on their relationship with God.

TALKING ABOUT GOD AS A JUDGE IN CANCER

In the metaphorical role as judge survivors believe God uses the breast cancer experience to get their attention. Whether it is to make them aware of the need to forgive or to change the way they live, by changing their priorities, God uses breast cancer to send a message. And the message God sends is about the need to change. Presented here are two survivor experiences of God as judge. In each, God reorients the survivor to focus on different concerns—misplaced priorities, inappropriate behaviors, and forgiveness. Breast cancer serves for both as God's vehicle to judge, nudging each survivor to adjust her way of thinking. Both adjust their behavior with the ultimate intent of improved psychosocial well-being.

Virginia Hudson—God Judges Personal Priorities

Virginia Hudson, a seventy-three-year-old retiree, is a fourteen-year breast cancer survivor. She first felt the lump in her breast three months after her annual physical examination, which included a clinical breast examination.[9] No lump was felt during her clinical exam. Diagnosed in 1988, Virginia had a mastectomy followed by chemotherapy. Virginia experienced several side effects from chemotherapy, including loss of appetite and an extreme distaste for certain foods and beverages she had previously enjoyed. The most serious side effect Virginia experienced following surgery and chemotherapy was that she developed an inability to swallow water. Hospitalized for severe dehydration, Virginia eventually regained the ability to swallow along with her appetite.

Supported throughout her treatment and aftercare by family and friends, especially her children, Virginia has been cancer free for almost two decades. Although she is grateful to be cancer free, she remains aware she could have a cancer recurrence in the future. Reflecting on her experience with cancer and life in general, Virginia sees unfortunate life events as something God does not necessarily intend for people to experience. Instead, she believes God uses negative situations to get people's attention. She thinks God helps people identify and develop better ways of living. Breast cancer, for her, represents this type of situation. God used this experience with breast cancer to act as Virginia's judge to lead her to a better and more purposeful life.

Virginia talks here about the issue of unfortunate events in life. Her expanded understanding of how God operates in people's lives, as evidence of her constructive theology, has brought some important revelations. As Virginia shares,

> When things happen to you and stuff, you think God has done something. I mean [you think that God] don't care and all that. But I have come to the conclusion, don't ask me cause I just read [the Bible], that God don't intend for you to have these things [cancer]. You bring them on your own self. I really think that. From the food you eat, the life you live, the things we do. He doesn't set the way. He sets the timing [of experiences]. I came to that conclusion and I really think that. I really believe that.
>
> At first [when I was diagnosed] I blamed my doctor because he didn't find it when I had the physical [three months before her diagnosis]. And I had a physical every year. But he didn't find it. And then I thought, "Well, God is mad at me or something." But he [God] didn't do it either [give me cancer]. And once you come to that conclusion [things make sense].
>
> That's just like you're getting saved. If it don't never come to your mind, people can talk from now on. You don't know what they're talking about. And that's the way this is. If you don't never do nothing [to think differently, then you remain the same]. [An example is] like my daughter sitting yonder smok-

> ing right now; see she's bringing it [misfortune] on herself. But she says she can't quit so she won't try.

Given her assessment of health and suffering as part of life, Virginia further added the following:

> You just have to take it [suffering]. People eat stuff and drink stuff and all that stuff. That's not [what God intends]. The Lord would be happier, I do believe, if you followed, if you was a nice healthy person and didn't have all of that suffering. But still when you come to the end of your life, you gonna leave this world. But you could be happy 'til then. You don't have to be suffering and everything. You bring that on through life. I really believe that. So I just accepted that it was going to come [suffering]. And it depended on the way I lived as to when and where.
>
> Even the worse you do helps you get to that end of your life. But I truly believe that if you live right, you live healthy, and you do the right things, you can be a healthy person. You have heard of people that just "fall dead," so to speak. And all the doctors can say is just "natural causes." Well they just got to the end of their lifeline, but they were just fine. That's what I think. I don't know when and still don't. My lifeline is running out. It might not even be from the cancer.

And finally, Virginia talks about what she has learned from her relationship with God. She relays how this has affected her understanding of breast cancer experience. Here Virginia talks about what God used breast cancer to make her aware of. For her, God judged her misplaced priorities regarding financial stability and economic self-sufficiency. Once Virginia could no longer work because of her breast cancer induced morbidity (i.e., lymphedema) she realized she could reorganize her finances and live comfortably. Virginia learned as a consequence of breast cancer that she could rely on God to supply her financial needs. As Virginia said,

> [Breast cancer] lets you take life more easily. I used to think that I was a workaholic. And when you work for state government, you are never going to get rich. But, you can make a living. Live decently. And I thought with all of this overtime and stuff, I could make it. And well now I'm just living on a little retirement and social security and I'm still making it. You really don't need all that. When you do extra work besides your regular job, you do extra things. You buy extra things. You get where you've got to have this extra money. But, you can make it without it. You'll make it without it. So once I found that out [I retired].

For Virginia, God used breast cancer to get her attention about particular aspects of living. Her reading of the Bible and related spiritual activities (i.e., prayer, meditation) allowed Virginia to continual talk with God. As a result,

Virginia developed an increasingly complex understanding of God as a metaphorical judge.

Early on, Virginia constructed God as a judge that sent breast cancer to her as a punishment or retribution for misdeeds. However upon greater reflection and study of the Bible, Virginia abandoned this construction of God as judge. She replaced this punitive construction of God with other ideas about God's functioning as judge. She likened her increasing understanding of God as judge and how a judge acts to that of the Christian conversion experience.

Christian conversion is an experience in which the convert undergoes a process of analytical reorganization, whereby they are transformed from a nonbeliever to a believer. Although the nonbeliever can be exposed to the beliefs and tenets of Christianity, the conversion of the believer only occurs when the believer changes his/her way of thinking. When the convert changes her/his thinking about God, likewise, they change. Through the conversion experience, a convert's relationship shifts from having a "relationship to" to instead having a "relationship with" God. Initially Virginia saw herself as being acted upon by God. She later came to see herself as being capable of acting in concert with God.

With Virginia's new understanding, God as a metaphorical judge functions not to punish, but instead to rehabilitate how she lives. God makes rehabilitation possible even in seemingly unfortunate circumstances. For Virginia rehabilitation is only afforded to people willing to admit their own limitations. Change happens when people desire to change. God for Virginia does not inflict suffering and misfortune. Instead, Virginia believes people bring negative (and positive) circumstances upon themselves through their health-related behaviors. She uses her daughter's inability to stop smoking to demonstrate where she believes, in part, the health locus of control for well-being actually resides. That is with the individual.

Yet, at the same time, Virginia believes people share responsibility for their health outcomes; she also believes that God plays a pivotal role. In the same way that a judge pronounces a sentence upon a convicted person, God controls the timing and duration of the sentence. For Virginia, God uses life events like breast cancer to underscore that some behavioral error has occurred. After these errors have been pointed out, for Virginia, locus of control shifts to external (i.e., God controlled) versus internal (i.e., survivor controlled).

Virginia believes God as judge used her breast cancer diagnosis to get her attention about her working overtime. Virginia, by her own admission, worked not because of financial need, but instead, to buy more things. God as judge used breast cancer to refocus Virginia's attentions on the source of her financial viability. Virginia's financial stability did not come from working more hours at her job. Her financial well-being came from her belief in

God's ability to totally supply her material needs. God as judge used Virginia's experience with breast cancer to show her that if she changed the way she thought about money she could live a much more contented life. As a judge, God taught Virginia that her well-being was contingent on living well with less.

Hattie Glover—God Administers and Commutes

Hattie Glover, a wife and mother, was diagnosed with breast cancer at the age of thirty-four.[10] She is a two-year breast cancer survivor. Hattie had a lumpectomy, followed by chemotherapy and radiation. Hattie endured before, during, and after breast cancer treatment what others might not have emotionally been able handle. Hattie's life has been punctuated by deaths, emotional upheavals, and new beginnings.

After a bitter divorce, Hattie rekindled a romantic relationship with a childhood friend. A few months later, she was diagnosed with breast cancer. This was quickly followed by chemotherapy. Four months after her diagnosis, her paternal grandmother passed. Shortly before her passing, Hattie got engaged. While undergoing chemotherapy, Hattie busily planned her wedding, slated for few months after she finished treatment. Once finished with chemotherapy, Hattie immediately started radiation. The week preceding her wedding, while still undergoing radiation therapy, her father passed. He had been scheduled to give her away during the ceremony.

Returning from her honeymoon, Hattie finished radiation. A short time after she finished radiation, Hattie found out she was pregnant during a routine physical. She had been pregnant during her cancer treatment. Neither she nor her oncology team had been aware of her pregnancy during her treatment. The week she delivered her baby, the plant she worked for closed. Left without severance pay, health benefits, or other compensatory benefits, Hattie is on state-sponsored Medicaid. Her children's medical coverage is covered by their fathers' insurance coverage. Despite everything that has happened in the two years since her diagnosis, Hattie considers herself fortunate to be able to ensure her family's basic health-care needs are covered. In the midst of all of these tumultuous circumstances, Hattie believes God was trying to get an important message to her.

Hattie believes breast cancer was God's way of nudging her to let go of painful past experiences. She has to let go of old wounds in order to live healthfully. God for Hattie sent a judgmental message not to hurt, but to help her. Hattie believes as part of constructive theology that because of her willingness to obey, God is continually commuting her sentence. As a metaphorical judge, God is turning all things around for Hattie's ultimate good. Hattie speaks at some length about her diagnosis,

> [When I was diagnosed with breast cancer] I was just mad, just mad. My cousin, he told me, "The reason you're going through this is because of Earl." Me and Earl, their father [the father of her older children]—we had a [bitter divorce]. I didn't forgive him. That's why God stepped in. And put it [breast cancer in my body]. I'll say put the cancer there. [It] was because I hadn't forgiven him. I mean you know you say you forgive and forget. But I hadn't forgiven him for all of the stuff; excuse me [expletive] that he took me through. Bottom line.

Hattie described the circumstances that fueled her animosity and resentment of her ex-husband. She explains the events that took place around their divorce. Her explanation of what happened locates for her the etiology of her breast cancer. As Hattie recalls,

> I was pregnant with Sarah [oldest daughter]. Divorcing him at the same time. He was going around saying that it wasn't his child. He said both of them weren't his children [her two oldest children]. [I was] hot [angry]. You see what I'm saying? Five-and-a-half years of marriage. That's why my cousin said that. He said, "That's why God has put this on you. But, he will only put on you what you can bear." And I still believe that to this day.

After her diagnosis, Hattie reflected on what her cousin said about the cause of her breast cancer. Hattie adopted what her cousin said as her own etiologic explanation for cancer. Once Hattie adopted this way of thinking about cancer, she modified her behavior, especially her resentment toward her ex-husband. When Hattie modified her behavior, she believes the dynamics of her breast cancer treatment also changed. To move beyond being angry with Earl, Hattie says,

> I just prayed about it. Prayed about it. And I said, "I don't have to be worried no more. I don't have to be with him no more."
>
> After I started forgiving Earl, the cancer went away. I'll tell you why [I believe this]. I only had to have two treatments [chemotherapy treatments]. And the doctor told me three or four. So you know God is still working, at that time. You know what I'm saying. Working.

As Hattie explains, God as judge continually worked to lessen the severity of her cancer treatment because of her willingness to forgive her ex-husband. Hattie's obedience to God changed her perspective toward her ex-husband. Her obedience was manifested through her prayers for her ex-husband. The results of her actions (i.e., fewer treatments, emotional peace) assure Hattie that she need no longer emotionally concern herself with him. Since her change in attitude, Hattie reports that her relationship with her ex-husband has changed. They have learned to be civil toward each other, especially regarding their children. This has consequently improved Hattie's psychosocial well-being. It has also improved her family's emotional well-being.

Hattie believes her psychosocial well-being and her family's well-being are the most important long-term benefits from her breast cancer experience. She has learned how to better handle situations that distress her. And Hattie has gained the confidence in God and herself to know if she faces other stressful situations again she can apply what she has learned to weather these psychosocial crises. Surviving breast cancer assures Hattie that she can succeed and thrive despite what happens. She believes her well-being ensures her family's well-being also.

Hattie thinks God acted as a judge in her breast cancer experience. Although she did not initially come to that conclusion on her own (i.e., her cousin's etiologic explanation), she came to strongly identify with this explanation. God as judge inflicted breast cancer on Hattie the same way a judge convicts a defendant. Hattie was sentenced with breast cancer because of repressed anger and resentment toward her ex-husband. She had not forgiven him for his psychological mistreatment. She told others she had forgiven him, but deep inside she knew that she had not. Further compounding resentment, Hattie admitted that she had lied to herself about actually forgiving her ex-husband. Resentments, un-forgiveness, anger, and un-truthfulness were the circumstances that caused Hattie's cancer. Into all of this pain, anger, and the disease/illness, Hattie believes God stepped in.

Breast cancer, as Hattie sees it, is judgment for her behavior. She underwent surgery and saw chemotherapy and radiation remained as other parts of her sentence. Like a person convicted and sentenced in the judicial system, Hattie believes she retained some power to affect the final outcome of her situation. Changing her situation's outcome required Hattie to be honest about what she believed "her crimes" to be (i.e., misbehavior). Coming clean with how she actually felt about her ex-husband, Hattie metaphorically threw herself upon the mercies of the court, evidenced through her reliance on prayer to communicate with God. When Hattie admitted her errors and sought to repay the debt she felt she owed (i.e., forgiving her ex-husband) God commuted her final sentence. Instead of having to go for three or four rounds of chemotherapy, Hattie only needed two. She attributes this change in her treatment course's duration to her willingness to obey what God called her to do. Hattie forgave her ex-husband. Consequently, God commuted her sentence.

For Hattie, God as judge continued to be lenient toward her. Chemotherapy and radiation usually create physiological conditions not conducive to conception and/or sustaining a pregnancy. Nevertheless, Hattie got pregnant while undergoing treatment. She delivered a healthy baby. God as judge in Hattie's breast cancer experience passed sentence and commuted her sentence. Hattie's sentence was commuted after she admitted her error and corrected her perceived misbehaviors.

GOD AS "LIBERATOR"

For some African American survivors, God is evidenced as a "liberator" in the cancer experience. God as liberator steps into situations to supernaturally heal cancer. As liberator, God also give survivors the wherewithal to endure cancer treatment. God liberates in several ways. As liberator God fortifies survivors' resolve so that they can cope with breast cancer. God also helps them adjust to whatever situations experiencing cancer brings.

Exercising their faith in God, survivors believe as part of their constructive theology that God will positively affect cancer situations and deliver them. God will, however it happens, successfully help them thorough breast cancer. Even after treatment, these cancer survivors believe God will sustain them in all circumstances they face, whether they are life threatening or not. God is a liberator available in all seasons and life situations. These African American cancer survivors believe God liberates them so they can share their cancer experiences with others. Survivors are liberated from cancer to function as living witnesses to God's abilities to heal those who believe.

Melba Scott—God Liberating a Living Witness

Melba Scott, a forty-eight-year-old wife and mother, is a successful administrator.[11] She is also an eight-year breast cancer survivor. After her diagnosis, Melba underwent a mastectomy, followed by chemotherapy. Some years later, she had reconstructive surgery to replace her breast. During this surgery, Melba underwent breast reduction surgery on her remaining breast to achieve symmetry between her breasts. She has been extremely satisfied with the results.

Melba came from humble beginnings in Mississippi. As a child she picked and chopped cotton to help financially support her family. Having risen through the ranks to attain her current position, Melba, as an educated, professional African American woman, has endured both racism and sexism as she climbed the corporate ladder. Struggle, therefore is not something Melba is unaccustomed. Melba appreciates what she has achieved. She is grateful for people she meets and help she has received. All of these experiences she credits to God. Melba believes that breast cancer is really no different from the other life experiences she has had because God has been with her.

When Melba underwent chemotherapy, she did not experience many of the common side effects of adjuvant treatment. She did get nauseated when she first began chemotherapy. Melba's hair did not fall out. She did not lose her appetite. Her hair kept growing and she kept having it chemically relaxed while she went through chemotherapy. Instead of losing weight, which often accompanies chemotherapy-induced appetite loss, Melba's appetite did not change and she even gained weight while having chemotherapy. Melba believes God sustained her during cancer treatment, making the seemingly impossible possible.

Beyond her own abiding faith that God would help her through breast cancer, others also tapped into God's liberation power on Melba's behalf. Melba's supporters drew from God's liberating power by praying. When she approached her church family about her situation, the church prayed for her deliverance. They prayed throughout her cancer treatment. The extent to which others prayed for her, Melba did not find out until after she finished chemotherapy. Others' faith and prayers, Melba believes, activated God's liberating power throughout breast cancer treatment and sustains her well-being.

Melba was initially reluctant to talk openly about her diagnosis. However, when she did, it felt as if a burden had been lifted,

> Initially I didn't talk about it [being diagnosed] and I do want you to know that. It was only after I had gone through my chemotherapy, six months of it as a matter of fact, and then I got up and did a testimony. None of my church family, at that point, knew.
>
> Once they found out, then I knew then everything would be all right. It was just a weight off my shoulders. And then I had people praying and fasting and all of that for me. So I'm just blessed, you know. And I talk about it now because I have a story to tell.
>
> What happened was the people in my Sunday school class knew. There were people at my job who knew. But, I just hadn't [told church members]. Just, like when I did the article [about her breast cancer experience], I had never done that. People that I knew knew from just me talking about it. But see I made up in my mind at that point [with the publication of the article] that God had given me an opportunity to beat this disease. That it was not just by fate that I was still here. That somebody had to be praying for me. What better place to give a testimony then in a church. And I did. I gave it. And once I gave [my testimony], it was a release off of me.
>
> I used to get emotional about it. But, it wasn't because I was sad about it. It was just that I was so happy about it and I'm able to control it a little bit better than I used to. But, every time that I talk about it, it helps somebody else.

Seeking affirmation of God's liberation in other cancer survivors' situations, Melba talks to other survivors. What Melba has learned from these exchanges with others diagnosed with cancer about spirituality, faith, and survivorship are part of a spirituality of survival Melba draws from. Melba uses this collective body of wisdom about God's liberation as symbol in the way Peters describes.[12] God's record of liberation for African American breast cancer survivors serves as a symbol that supports theological faithfulness. As Melba says,

> Everybody that I've talked to, who has had any form of cancer, whether it be breast cancer or whatever else, they say what got them through was faith based. They talked about it at church. They had their ministers and they had their friends pray for them. I had a prayer chain of people who prayed for me every day. Now it's amazing that I never requested this. Someone requested it for me. And I only found it out after the fact.
>
> And when I get up and talk about people doing things for me, I tell them to call my name, I want you to say, "Melba Scott" because I believe it. Irregardless of what I've gone through, I just think prayer, it works.
>
> And I believe that there are people who are faith based who are good prayer warriors, as you call them, and as we know them. They had a lot to do with me being healed. And I know that for a fact.

Melba believes in the power of prayer to access God's liberation power. Melba talks about how this liberating power was accessed for her during a church service. The Sunday Melba gave her initial testimony in church, she remembers,

> My pastor—we talked about this [cancer diagnosis and treatment]. And then he claimed the victory with all of us. He claimed victory [healing and resolution for] my cancer. He put the oil [on me, as part of laying on of hands] and did his blessing. I was through with it [worrying about treatment and surviving].

For Melba, God's liberation has happened in several ways. Primarily, she is liberated from worrying about her cancer survivorship. Melba shares how she felt after her initial testimony in her church,

> I wasn't worried about a thing because I knew I was going to be okay. And I have been. I just think that [was what helped heal me]. I just think that. And I don't know how nobody can't [believe]. How they cannot even think that [this helped to heal me]. Sure man and medicine can do a lot for you. But, they don't know everything. I just think God has something to do with this.

Recalling the circumstances of another Sunday church service, following her initial cancer testimony in church, Melba recalls,

> [This Sunday] I got up in church and I talked about the fact that I was going back for chemotherapy. I had been through six months of chemotherapy and I was going back for my check-ups. I just went through the whole trial. I had to go every three months for my chest x-rays. And after so many years, I go once a year. And I got up and said, "I'm going in on Wednesday." And I got back the next Sunday and told them, "I told you all the wrong date."

> Then the pastors' wife said to me, "Melba, I fasted [for you]. I know it's going to be fine for you." And then someone else said, "I did this for you." But, I did not know.
>
> Now let me tell you this. See, I was sick this whole time. I only knew when I got back to my church home that people had done all of these things for me. Because I didn't know that they had prayed for me. And one guy said, "You all have been truly blessed, honey, because the whole church has prayed for you."

Melba believes her experiences during cancer treatment and afterward evidence God's liberating power. She believes her liberation from side effects common with breast cancer treatment happened because of others' petitions to God for liberating power on her behalf. What others do on her behalf is important. However, Melba believes she also has a role to play. Although others pray for her, she also prays for herself. Collectively, these acts of faith are linked together. Melba says the following about these matters,

> I know it had to have been something because I just didn't have any problems. I just didn't. I mean I was expecting all of these things to happen to me and it didn't. It just didn't. And I knew somebody had to pray for me. And that's what happened. And I just believe and I continue to say that I want somebody to pray for me. No. I don't just want you to pray for me. I want you to pray with me.

In Melba's situation, God is revealed as a liberator. God healed her body of cancer. God's liberation came in several ways. Melba used conventional biomedical treatment for breast cancer to heal. But for Melba, surgery and chemotherapy were not enough. Melba needed other healing interventions to support her well-being.

For Melba, biomedicine provides technologies and human expertise to ameliorate breast cancer symptoms; however, these technologies and expertise by themselves cannot eliminate and/or prevent cancer. Melba believes God works through various strategies to heal and deliver survivors from breast cancer. Pastoral consultation, anointing with oil as a religious ritual, specific requests made for divine healing (i.e., claiming the "victory" over the disease/illness), fasting, and prayer all work collectively to support Melba's well-being. Each is part of a network of healing God manifests liberation through for Melba.

Using her faith, particularly through prayer and evidenced in faith about her divine healing, Melba taps into God's liberating power to heal her breast cancer. Melba links her faith with that of others to ensure and sustain positive well-being. These acts of faith (e.g., anointing with oil, fasting, organized prayer chains) and biomedical treatment, which for Melba requires faith to believe in its efficacy, all reveal God's liberating power in Melba's breast cancer experience.

Melba's blessing of well-being requires her to share her story with others, so they too might be encouraged and their faith affirmed in God. Melba's testifying is demonstrative of Gilkes's "process of critical remembering," whereby the testimony of individual triumph of over adversities is transformed into a prophetic resource for the larger community.[13] This testimony becomes a resource, part of the constructive theology's tradition that demonstrates to others strategies of how to use faith in God and personal struggles to survive.

It is interesting that Melba's (re)telling of her story provides continual opportunities to reaffirm for her God as liberator. When she speaks to other cancer survivors, Melba says she is repeatedly told faith-based practices and beliefs are what sustain others throughout their cancer experiences. When Melba talks about "faith-based efforts," she does not think this is a domain exclusive to Christian believers. In Melba's cancer experience, her liberation from breast cancer comes from God. For others, she believes their liberation can come through faith in some other manifestation of a higher being or power. For Melba's theology, what is most critical to healing is one's appreciation that liberation comes from an external source, one not limited to one's personal power or abilities.

When Melba talks about God, this talking is not limited only to ritualized religious activities and/or a formal institutional structure. Some specific healing activities did happen for Melba during church worship activities (i.e., services). However, God's liberation is not limited to these situations. Melba believes God's healing and liberating power happen through an ongoing communicative relationship with God. She accesses God's liberation through faith. Absence of cancer in Melba's body is evidence of God's liberation. God liberates Melba from breast cancer so she can witness that fact to others. Melba is liberated by God to serve others through her testimony.

Krystal Young—God's Liberation in Mysterious Ways

Krystal Young is a thirty-something married minister who, after her diagnosis, underwent a lumpectomy followed by radiation.[14] After diagnosis, Krystal looked for answers about why she had to be diagnosed with breast cancer. She posed her questions about how to maneuver through breast cancer to God. When all other support systems failed or gave her less than helpful advice, Krystal talked to God and listened for God's response.

Seeking God's direction, Krystal used scripture as a basis for theological understanding. Particular revelation came through the biblical story of Job. In scripture, Krystal received assurance she is divinely healed from breast cancer. Although confident she is healed, God nevertheless told Krystal to proceed with biomedical care. At first, she believed God's commands did not make sense. Later however Krystal came to understand why God commanded her to act in seemingly contradictory ways to achieve healing. God required Krystal undergo biomedical treatment so that there might be visible proof of her healing. Proof of her divine healing would be evidenced by her mammography films, which showed she was cancer free. Krystal believed God wanted to reveal to her that she had been and would continue to be liberated from cancer.

Setting the stage for God's presence as a liberator, Krystal talked about her breast cancer diagnosis and the emotional turmoil that it brought. Krystal shared in detail the circumstances surrounding her diagnosis and her treatment decision-making. Krystal remembers the events this way:

> In December of '06 [2006] I went in on Friday to have the mammogram done. They got the results Monday. Monday evening they called me and said that they had gotten my results back and they were suspicious. By Friday I was in the doctor's office. They had already set up, scheduled, my exam with what I found out later to be a breast cancer specialist. But they didn't say that. They just said to me, "We have a breast specialist, who needs to talk with you about your mammogram." So then I went in. He then set me up the following week for a biopsy. To see how it was looking. And he thought it might have been cystic milk glands. That [assessment] made me feel more comfortable with the first one [suspicious mammography results].
>
> When it came back, he said to me that I had cancer. And that was, you know—that word just shook me up. And not only did he tell me I had cancer, but the entire tip of the biopsy was completely involved. And he indicated that he was suspicious that my entire chest wall might be involved. And with him being a specialist, of course that really scared me.

Krystal, as she admits, was scared and shaken up by her breast cancer diagnosis. Her oncologist felt he was helping her by preparing her for the possibility of metastasis (cancer spreading to other areas of the body). However, instead of allying Krystal's fears, the diagnosis only increased her anxiety about her prognosis. Krystal needed advice and reassurance. She turned to God and her family for support. This is what Krystal shared about what happened after her diagnosis:

> At this time [after the diagnosis], even though I had prayed about [it], I was very serious in my prayer about it. I went to God and demanded an answer as to why I was having to deal with this. And then there were people talking to me, family members, whom I could depend on to tell them anything. They would help me. They would pull me through whatever obstacles I was going through. And all of my support systems started to break down in between the two surgeries [biopsy and lumpectomy].
>
> Their recommendations to me were that I get a second opinion. Secondly, that I not let him cut on me again. Because once the air hits it, then it would

> spread all over my body. So I was really not getting support. At this point the only person that I had to turn to was God.

Instead of receiving the support she needed to make the most informed treatment decisions, Krystal received conflicting recommendations from her family. Their advice did not mitigate her fears about her breast cancer diagnosis. Instead, their advice made her even more nervous and indecisive about how to proceed with treatment. To make the best treatment decision possible, Krystal finally decided to rely solely on God for guidance. Turning to God for direction, Krystal recalls the specifics of her prayer/conversation with God. As she reflects,

> In my prayer to him [God], he revealed to me that I [should look in the Bible]. He took my mind to the book of Job and said, "Read that." I went to the book of Job and read it. Understanding that Job was upright. And it [his suffering] was [as a result of] nothing Job did. He was "perfect and upright" is what God used for him [to describe Job].
>
> I did not consider myself to be perfect and completely upright. Even though my relationship with God [had improved] because I had just gone into the ministry months before and preached my first sermon. At this time I thought, "I'm more righteous than I've ever been." And yet this kind of thing happened to me. So I don't understand it. And so when he told me to read the book of Job, like, "Job will tell you." And when I went and read the book I basically put my name where "Job" was and put myself in his exact predicament. I was losing family members. Even though they were not dying, they were being lost to me mentally and spiritually, as a support group. I understood what that meant to be by yourself.
>
> And so right then I said, "Thank you, God." And I said, "God, I don't understand all of this. All of this is too much for me to handle. I read and understood about Job. But, [questioning God], "You weren't cutting on Job's body. You had put sores [on Job's body]. So what am I to do?"

Reading the biblical book of Job, Krystal received a revelation of healing. God spoke through Job's experience to show Krystal that God had liberated Job from his suffering and sickness. God intended to do the same for her. Krystal shared how God revealed God's intent to serve as her liberator.

> After I had read the book of Job, I felt this sense of peace come over me and I could hear God saying, "You're healed." And at that point, I just jumped up. That was what I had wanted to hear. I heard what I wanted to hear on Monday before I went in for surgery. So shortly after that the doctor called me [about whether she wanted reconstruction during her lumpectomy]. When the doctor called, I said, "Okay. Let me think about it and I'll call you back." After I got off the phone I said, "God, you said I was healed. And now he's telling me about an implant. What do I tell him?"

> And God spoke and said, "You won't need it." And I said, "Okay." I said, "Okay." So I went back and called the doctor right back. "I won't need the implant." You can let your friend go home, in other words.

As Krystal understands God's liberation revealed to her in scripture, she is healed from cancer. Although she is healed, she still underwent surgery. Even in this, God orchestrated the events of Krystal's surgery to make reconstruction unnecessary.

Krystal later recalled the day of her lumpectomy. She was pleased that God had revealed her liberation (i.e., healing) from cancer. Nevertheless, Krystal was still perturbed with God. Why go undergo surgery if her healing had already taken place. Krystal wanted an answer from God about this. But God seemed unwilling to offer an answer. The circumstances of this liberating healing did not seem to make sense. Krystal remembers,

> When I got up early the next morning [the day following her healing revelation] I was focused on getting dressed and everything. And my prayer really was not that focused a prayer. It was like, "Let's get this show on the road." It was very casual.
>
> I was really perturbed with God at this point because I'm not understanding him. And we're not half speaking at this point. And so at this point on the way to the hospital, my husband is quiet and my daughter is quiet. They're in the car with me. And in the stillness I said to God, "God, you are having me to go through this, which I don't understand. Since you are having me to go through it, I don't have time for this hospital delay [surgery and recovery] so take me through this surgery successfully. Let your angels encamp around me. And get me up quickly because I have something to do. I am too busy for this." And so that was the end of prayer. "Thank you, God."

Still somewhat upset with God, Krystal continued to talk to God, asking God to intercede during her surgery. Krystal specifically asked God to manifest God's liberating presence during surgery in three ways. First, she asked God to bring her through the surgery successfully—liberate her by allowing the surgeons to successfully remove the tumor. Next, Krystal asked God to free her by providing angels to comfort and attend to her appropriately during surgery. Krystal called upon the presence of angels, as God's messengers, to protect her from potentially negative outcomes (i.e., death or pain during surgery). She also asked for these angels to usher her into positive ones outcomes (i.e., successful tumor removal, cancer survival). And finally, Krystal evoked God's liberating power by asking God to heal her quickly from surgery so she might return quickly to her normal activities.

At the time of her prayer, Krystal felt she was going through the motions of evoking God's liberation. She was perturbed and frustrated by the turn of events in her life. Krystal's attention was on getting through the surgery. Although she knew God was present, she did not believe God heard or would answer her hasty and half-hearted requests. But, even though she did not realize it at the time, God did respond to her prayer. This is how Krystal recalls the specifics of her surgery,

> By this time we are at the hospital. I go into the hospital. They go through all of the preoperative stuff, checking in and all. And the doctor comes in. The nurses are just extremely kind, which was kind of unusual. But I didn't connect it to my prayer, at this point. They were just extremely nice this early in the morning. Everybody.
>
> And the doctor came in with the anesthesiologist. She greeted me. And then she said, "This is my assistant. We are here to make sure that you don't feel any pain. We have brought enough medication [to insure this]." She said, "We are prepared to keep you under as long as we need to and you won't feel a thing." And they started the IV into my arm at that time.

The pleasant and reassuring disposition of the medical personnel helped to dispel some of Krystal's fears and frustrations about surgery. Krystal received further supportive care from another member of her medical team. Krystal described what her surgeon did to further calm her after the intravenous drip started.

> The doctor said, "You are going to be fine." He [the surgeon] said, "Do you mind if I pray with you?" I said, "No, not at all." You know? So he prayed a fairly short prayer. And I remember him saying on the end, "God, don't allow me to do any more than I have to do." And so that just stuck out in my mind like, "Listen." And it clicked, you know. And with that she [the anesthesiologist] started the medication in. And that's all I remember.

After surgery, Krystal recalled at first feeling as if she had died during the operation. Everything in the operating room seemed surreal. In order to assure herself that she had not died, Krystal performed her own reality check. She remembers the circumstances this way:

> When I came to in the recovery room I could hear them saying, "She's awake!" And they all came and got around my bed. There were male and female nurses. They all had on white. And when I first saw them, the room just sparkled. And I thought, "Oh, my God. I'm in heaven!" They came over and started talking to me and patting me like, "You awake?" And I guess I was kind of going in and out. [They asked,] "How are you feeling? You feel any pain?" and all this. And I was afraid to look down because [I knew part of my breast had been removed]. And then I realized, "Reality check. Okay. You are still here!" But I still didn't connect the guardian angel part of my prayer, at that time.
>
> And then they came around me. And they just said, "You came through it beautifully." And I said, "What do you mean, 'beautifully'?" I am afraid to look at my breast.

> My husband came in he said, "You're fine." From the smile on his face I knew that everything was okay.
>
> The doctor came in and told me that he had sent my biopsy to the lab and they had kept me under while they sent it to the lab to be cultured. "We got a clean module. There's no[thing], except for the spot that we went down into."
>
> "We went down into a cluster of three very small pearl-sized growths." And he said, "I took out enough tissue this time to make sure that we had a clean module. There is nothing in the module. The module is clear all the way around." So obviously it was just those three little small ones. He said, "I'll be sending it to the lab. In four days if there is any more growth then we'll have to come back and do the surgery again."
>
> So I said, "Okay." At this point, I thought, "You got a clean module; I'm taking that. That's the report I want to hear because I've been healed."

Although the healing circumstances did not happen the way Krystal expected, she came away with the result she desired. She was cancer free. The cancer had not spread to other areas of her body, but was localized to her breast. Her prognosis for long-term survival was favorable. Krystal received the liberation from cancer she desired.

Krystal later reflects on how God further revealed God's self as liberator in her breast cancer experience. Her divine revelation through the story of Job, her prayer, the surgery, and the caring and supportive actions of her health-care providers had all been for a reason. The reason was to ensure her healing. Krystal shared this about God's revelation to her as a liberator:

> I truly believe that at the time when I finished the book of Job in one day [I was healed]. I sat there and I literally ate that book of Job for breakfast, lunch, and dinner. I just sat there all day. I just sat reading. By the time I finished, I could understand clearly. And there, that brought about the peace in my spirit. I also believed because I could feel a sensation as I was praying thanking God for helping me to understand what he had to do with Job [by allowing him to suffer].
>
> A couple of months or so after I had gone through all my treatment and everything, the Lord revealed something to me. I was just praying one day. And I said, "I didn't understand why you did that? [Required me undergo a lumpectomy] But, it's okay." He said, "Now you have before and after pictures. Now you have a stronger testimony."
>
> Every time I go to the doctor and they say, "No cancer," healing is still going on, you know. But, if I didn't have those pictures. I had a picture showing that I did in fact have cancer. But since then, every time I go back it shows that you are still healed. You were healed. You are being healed. You will be healed, you know. So it's a continuous process. So every time, it's just a matter of where are you in the process, you know [that I am healed]. So I just thank God for what he has done.

Krystal believes God liberated her from breast cancer. Each time she goes for a mammogram and comes away with a positive result, Krystal's faith in

God is strengthened. She is continually reassured that God is perpetually healing her body to prevent recurrence. God's presence as a liberator is an ongoing process of restoring Krystal's body and emotions.

In Krystal's experience with breast cancer, God revealed aspects of God's nature as a divine liberator. God revealed this particularly to her through biblical scripture—namely, the story of Job. God used the book of Job to talk to Krystal about her breast cancer diagnosis and treatment. Krystal's experience, along with scripture served as tools to shape her constructive theology. She understood God's nature to be revealed in scripture and evidenced in her cancer treatment.

God as liberator became most obvious after Krystal exhausted all of seemingly available avenues of support and advice. God became her liberator once she focused complete attention on seeking and listening for God's guidance. When all others failed, Krystal decided to talk to God. As she had hoped, God did not fail to talk to her about her most urgent needs—emotional comfort and advice about surgery.

After reading the Biblical story of Job, the man who lost everything and regained health and prosperity at the end of his test of faith, Krystal felt a sense of peace about her own situation. While she was feeling peaceful, God spoke to Krystal, revealing God's intentions for her well-being. God communicated what she most wanted to hear—she was healed from breast cancer. God liberated Krystal from what she feared most, cancer and its spread throughout her body.

Although God liberated Krystal from breast cancer, nevertheless, God instructed her to go through with having surgery and radiation. These instructions seemed to contradict the divine revelation of healing Krystal received. As Krystal believes, God desired to liberate (i.e., heal) more than just her body. God also wanted to liberate Krystal from the fear of cancer recurrence. This is where God's liberating nature became even more important for Krystal's well-being.

Unclear about why God would require her to have a lumpectomy after she received her healing revelation, Krystal admits she was initially angry with God. She thought God was being unreasonable. Why go through with surgeries if I have already been healed? This was the question Krystal posed to God. Continuing with surgery did not seem to make logical sense.

At the same time Krystal talked to God, God seemed resolute not to offer any explanations for why she needed surgery. Krystal had received instructions and was expected to comply. The fact that God's decisions did not make sense to Krystal seemed to be of little consequence to God in Krystal's estimation. Krystal's compliance did not hinge upon her understanding God's motivations or actions. God's actions, as Krystal reconciled them as part of her theology, at times defy human comprehension and reasoning. Hers was this kind of situation.

After making peace with what had happened, God revealed God's self again to Krystal as a liberator. This happened only after Krystal stilled herself to hear what God wished to reveal. God talked back to Krystal revealing the surgery, radiation, and subsequent screenings were intended for a purpose she had not considered. Instead of proving she had cancer, each of these procedures was intended to affirm that she was healed from cancer. The cancer that had been present was no longer in her breast. Nor was cancer anywhere else in her body. God liberated Krystal from breast cancer. The pictures are her proof.

Each screening Krystal undergoes thereafter reconfirms that God liberated her from cancer. Every test indicating she is cancer free renews her faith in God as a liberator and supports her constructive theology. Each medical encounter further strengthens her testimony of God's liberating power to heal. Krystal, in turn becomes a living witness of God's abilities to liberate by healing. Her story and the pictures support her belief in God and enhance her well-being.

Some of the clearest opportunities to see how God fully operates in the lives of African American breast cancer survivors are in times of emotional and/or psychological crisis. Breast cancer provides such opportunities for survivors. To better understand these phenomena, Brown-Douglass's pneumatology as the study of the Holy Spirit has been used.[15] Interpreted as the operational roles of God in the lives of African American breast cancer survivors, God's nature and power are evidenced as two prevailing metaphors, God as judge and liberator.

God as a metaphorical judge does not inflict women with breast cancer to hurt them. Instead, survivors as part of their constructive theology, interpret God as using breast cancer the way a judge might with a defendant—to send a message. God informs survivors that rehabilitation is necessary. As a judge, God uses breast cancer to help survivors take the actions necessary to alter their living. God helps survivors make their lives less complicated, stressful, and more personally rewarding and fulfilling. God as judge seeks to help survivors turn their lives around so that they can achieve well-being.

As a metaphorical liberator, God also desires the best for survivors. Instead of indicating that survivors make particular behavioral changes, God liberates survivors for other reasons. Namely God liberates survivors to strengthen their testimonies about God's abilities to heal. Even as a liberator, God's liberation is complex. Sometimes, God completely heals survivors by removing cancer from their bodies. At others, cancer survivors believe God works through others (i.e., physicians, church members) to ensure cancer survivors' healing and emotional restoration is complete. Still other survivors believe maintaining emotional balance and/or exuding confidence about long-term survival evidence God's liberating power, which sustains them through breast cancer.

African American breast cancer survivors' constructive theology serves at least two important functions. First, understanding God's roles and nature in the breast cancer experiences helps cancer survivors makes sense of the disease/illness situation. God's functions offer explanations about why survivors developed breast cancer. God's roles suggest to survivors the reasons why treatment and their attendant emotional upheavals are necessary. God's roles, as part of African American breast cancer survivors' constructive theology, provide analytical order in the midst of breast cancer's ensuing physical and psychosocial disorder.

African American breast cancer survivors' constructive theology decreases their anxiety after diagnosis and during treatment. These survivors, like all human beings, crave the ability to predict what is to come. Possessing this ability helps facilitate survivors' coping and adaptation. African American breast cancer survivors' constructive theology provides this. While their individual experiences of breast cancer may defy prediction, God's roles and nature provide predictive stability about survivors' futures.

The disease/illness of breast cancer assuredly comes with uncertainty. Yet, for these survivors, God stands at the center of their shifting health circumstances. God's ways might not always be predictable, but God's unwavering presence in survivors' experiences is constant. The consistency of God's presence supports African American breast cancer survivors' well-being. God provides explanation and creates order, making for them a way out of no way.

NOTES

1. Lindbeck, George. (2009). *The Nature of Doctrine: Religion and Theology in the Post-liberal Age.* Louisville, KY: Westminster John Knox Press.
2. Park, C., and Folkman, S. (1997). "Meaning in the Context of Stress and Coping." *Review of General Psychology, 1*, 115–144.
3. Cone, James. (2003). *God of the Oppressed.* Maryknoll, NY: Orbis Books; and Cone, James. (1997). *Black Theology & Black Power.* Maryknoll, NY: Orbis Books.
4. Peters, Ted. (2015). *God—The World's Future: Systematic Theology for the New Era.* Minneapolis: Augsburg Fortress.
5. Brown-Douglass, K. (1993). "Womanist Theology: What Is Its Relationship to Black Theology?" In Cone, James, and G. Wilmore (Eds.), *Black Theology: A Documentary History*, vol. 2, *1980–1992*, 290–299. Maryknoll, NY: Orbis Books.
6. Ibid.
7. Ibid.
8. Brown-Douglass, K. (1995). *The Black Christ.* Maryknoll, NY: Orbis Books.
9. Virginia Hudson is a pseudonym and details about her life are fictionalized to protect her privacy.
10. Hattie Glover is a pseudonym and details about her life have been fictionalized.
11. Melba Scott is a pseudonym and details about her life have been fictionalized.
12. Peters. *God—The World's Future: Systematic Theology for the New Era.*

13. Gilkes, C. *If It Wasn't for the Women: Black Women's Experience and Womanist Culture in Church and Community.* Maryknoll, NY: Orbis Books, 2001, 182.
14. Krystal Young is a pseudonym and details about her life have been fictionalized.
15. Brown-Douglass, *The Black Christ.*

Chapter Two

The Power of Black Women's Cancer Testimonies

Socially marginalized people often do their best theorizing in their cultural productions. Testimonies, diaries, letters, and other texts reflect what African American women think and how they feel. This is exemplified in Black women's scholarship[1] and in cancer survivors' journals.[2] Cancer testimonies, as cultural productions, reflect what African American breast cancer survivors think about themselves and cancer.[3] As embodied "texts," African American breast cancer survivors' testimonies particularly reflect ideas about cancer that come from their lived experiences with the disease.

Black breast cancer survivors' testimonies, particularly those about how they have been transformed as a consequence of cancer, have a logical structure. They usually include signs and symbols as important life markers.[4] Cancer testimonies in this way serve as "webs of significance" African American breast cancer survivors spin to make sense of their everyday lives.[5] In this study, observing, participating in, listening to, analyzing and interpreting, reflecting upon, and describing cancer survivors' testimonies have brought these webs of significance forward.

For these survivors, God is an important cultural symbol. God represents comfort, sustenance, care, purpose, healing, and loving correction to survivors. God also represents transformation and change. As a cultural symbol, God encompasses several ideas Black cancer survivors see as important to their hope and well-being. Testimony is the way survivors voice where and how God functions in their lives and why God is important to their survivorship. Talking about God is one important component of the thick description of African American cancer testimonies and the breast cancer experience.

Another important component of cancer testimonies is their actual telling or the act of testifying. Testifying is an essential part of well-being for many

African American breast cancer survivors. Openly talking about what they experience is often cathartic. A survivor's cancer testimony, when shared with others, feels therapeutic. Testifying about cancer as an intentional act is personally helpful to many cancer survivors. Yet, some survivors also believe their testimonies benefit others too. They believe their personal accounts of breast cancer give others hope, especially those facing difficult life situations. In these instances, their testifying offers therapeutic support for others' well-being.

When African American breast cancer survivors testify about cancer, doing so is not arbitrary. Testifying, as an act that supports well-being, is part of the tradition of the black religious experience and the Black Church.[6] Moore defines testifying as a "confessional tradition within the black religious experience . . . used in reference to the 'subjective' self-representations, interpretation and experiences recounted in autobiographical narratives and related materials."[7] Historically in the Black Church parishioners testified publicly about their challenges. As a part of the patterned structure of these testimonies, parishioners also acknowledged God's presence in trying situations in unexpected and even miraculous ways. Listeners, in turn, became witnesses to the testimonies they heard, finding points of commonality in their own lives, which further affirmed God's presence in both the tellers' and listeners' lives.

Parishioners' testimonies not only attested to God's transcendent presence and power at work, but also to the reality of life challenges. Testimonies in the Black Church reflected the ongoing interplay between God, people, and life. No matter how dire the situation, parishioners' testimonies included an undercurrent of hope. Despite what happened in life, God always prevailed. Testimonies in the Black Church tradition had the obvious benefit of steadying the teller's faith in God. Parishioners testified not because they felt defeated. They gave testimonies because they believed they would overcome no matter what the circumstance.

These testimonies had an additional benefit. Their telling strengthened the faith of those hearing them. Hearers came to believe God's possibilities for their own lives. Testimonies built up parishioners' faith. Testimonies shared publicly became part of an ongoing chronicle across time of what God can do. They also functioned as important tools for faith formation and community building. Tellers and hearers identified with each other through their testimonies and encouraged each other. Testifying, in turn, cultivated well-being.

Contemporary African American breast cancer survivors have adopted testifying about breast cancer as a wellness strategy. Instead of keeping the lived experience of breast cancer to themselves, many choose to tell their stories publicly. They testify about breast cancer and the challenges it creates for their lives. They also testify about God. At times, survivors testify for emotional release. Others are more strategic about how they use their testimonies. Some use them intentionally to help others. Breast cancer testimonies consequently benefit well-being on two fronts—personal well-being and community well-being.

Cancer survivors' testimonies are similar to what Kleinman calls *illness narratives*.[8] These stories about the etiology of disease and what people think about illness have been studied extensively in medical anthropology. More recent work in the area of narrative medicine similarly examines patients' stories and illness experiences.[9] Cancer testimonies shared in the context of medicine are usually intended to benefit diagnosis and treatment. By listening carefully to patients' narratives, health-care providers gain deeper insight about their patients. By listening to these testimonies, health-care providers increase their cultural sensitivity to patients' social contexts and histories, which presumably translates into improved treatment delivery and medical adherence.

African American breast cancer survivors' testimonies however are not exclusive to their encounters with health-care providers. These survivors' testimonies do not just benefit their diagnosis and treatment. African American breast cancer survivors tell their stories about breast cancer and what it teaches them to first bolster their faith. Testimonies serve as records of tests cancer survivors have experienced and ultimately won. Cancer survivors' testimonies sometimes acknowledge mistakes survivors believe they make and how these mistakes lead to or impact their breast cancers. Testimonies, while at times acknowledging survivors' perceived mistakes, never talk about them as insurmountable. Cancer survivors' testimonies generally reflect a hope in a future good, which survivors claim as having been achieved in the present. Instead of final outcomes, mistakes for African American breast cancer survivors serve as opportunities to learn more about themselves and God. African American cancer survivors reframe in their testimonies what seems bad, as being for their good.

Krystal Young's testimony provides an example of the structure of African American breast cancer survivors' testimonies and the webs of significance they create for cancer survivors. She frames breast cancer as an opportunity for good. Krystal's painful past experiences, as she discovered, were not intended to hurt her, but to help her reach others. Testifying has become a way of life for Krystal, a particularly effective way to maintain her health and well-being.

KRYSTAL YOUNG—TESTIFYING ABOUT CANCER

Krystal Young is a successful wife and mother.[10] As a minister, Krystal counsels sex workers and women who want to turn their lives around. She ministers to their needs by sharing her testimony as a breast cancer survivor. Although the lives of women who exchange sex for money and that of a minister and breast cancer survivors seem like worlds apart, Krystal knows otherwise. She understands that people sometimes respond to painful situations in self-destructive ways. Krystal has learned how to connect to people she otherwise would not be able to relate to as a consequence of having breast cancer.

A transformational part of Krystal's survivorship has been her cancer testimony. Her cancer testimony did not begin with her diagnosis and treatment. No, in many ways her cancer testimony predated her actual diagnosis. What she experienced before cancer shaped what she learned from breast cancer. Earlier experiences and the revelation she received about those experiences are interwoven into her cancer testimony. When Krystal was in college, her college sweetheart and fiancé cheated on her. She felt betrayed. The emotional trauma she experienced caused her to detach from her feelings. Rather than focus on her own pain, Krystal turned her attention to filling her time with other activities,

> To make sure that I was focused I disconnected myself emotionally. I had no feelings. I disconnected myself emotionally. I started to write things down so it would remind me to stay focused. I filled my schedule such that I would not have time to think and to ponder on things. If I stayed busy I didn't have time to think about me. And I also did things for other people. I made myself so busy with other people. And that kept me going. And so I didn't have to focus on me. My needs were insignificant.

To cope, Krystal had a string of superficial romantic relationships. This was her way of getting back at her ex-fiancé and God for her pain. When Krystal later married, she also became a mother and a minister. She suppressed all of the earlier feelings she had, burying them deep in her psyche.

When Krystal went into ministry a short while before her cancer diagnosis, she asked God to reveal whom she was to minister to. What God revealed to her was startling. She was called to counsel sex workers.

> I just started praying and asking God to reveal to me what ministry he had for me. "I don't want to miss anything you have for me. What ministry do you have for me?" And he showed me. He said, "You remember the whore on the street that you passed?" And I thought about going down on Rayburn Street at that time and seeing the prostitutes on the street. He said, "Those are the women that I want you to minister to." I thought, "Okay. Alright." I get this bigheaded attitude like, "Okay. Let me go down here and clean Rayburn Street up. First woman I see out here I'm going to tell her about herself. Filthy, nasty thing." But before I could go there, he said, "Because you can identify with her." And I said, "What?" I had been married at that time twenty-five years. Been completely faithful to my marriage. I thought, "What is he talking

> about?" Like, "Who? How can I relate to her? I'm better than this! I don't know anything about what goes on in their minds."

Krystal did not believe she shared anything in common with sex workers. Yet, when she underwent cancer treatment, her connection to these women became more apparent. What connected her and these women was suppressed emotional pain. As she recalls,

> [During radiation] he [God] gave me flashbacks. And that [the experience of breast cancer] was the first time I had been able to deal with that. That stuff was so painful. I had suppressed that back into my memory. I had read stories about people having stuff happen to them and they go under truth serum. And it's [memories] brought back up. And I had thought that's a bunch of bull, you know. But, this was so deeply suppressed—the hurt, anger, and the pain. It [college] was the most painful years of my life.

It was not until her cancer diagnosis and treatment that those long held feelings of betrayal, anger and hurt resurfaced. Krystal's feelings were connected to her cancer testimony.

During breast cancer treatment, Krystal's feelings of betrayal by God resurfaced. As she sought answers from God about why she had breast cancer, Krystal says God began to reveal the connection between her and the sex workers she ministers to. What they shared in common was pain and the ability to detach from it, particularly through sexual encounters.

> [Through my memories] God had said to me, "The only difference between you and her, them, is that you're cleaner. You picked yours from church, from your job, from other places. You didn't go out in the street. But, you didn't care who it really was." And the Lord just showed me, "I cleaned you up." [God continued,] "I gave you a husband and I gave you a child. I gave you a lifestyle that a lot of people envy. So I can do the same thing for them. That's all I want for you to do." [God said,] "I'm not doing this to beat you up. I'm doing this so you can go out there and say, "You don't have to do this. I know what you are feeling. I know your hurts. I know your pain." So with all of this, even with the breast cancer, all of this has been for ministry.

Krystal's testimony reflects her innermost thoughts and feelings. It also indicates how she saw herself. Her testimony, as those of many African American breast cancer survivors, reflects God's continued presence in her life. Krystal's cancer testimony functions as a map of her life before, during, and since breast cancer.

Krystal's cancer testimony is impactful by itself. However what gives it added weight is that she freely shares it with others. Krystal regularly testifies about having had breast cancer because it helps her connect to others. Seeing her as a survivor helps others believe they can survive challenges they face. Testifying is an essential component of a cancer testimony for African American breast cancer survivors. For what is the point of passing a test if you are not willing to tell others that you passed it. Testifying supports these cancer survivors' well-being. As Krystal says,

> All of this is for ministry and for a testimony. That's why I share it so much. I've talked to some other people who have gone through these kinds of situations. They ask me, "How can you talk about that kind of stuff? How can you still talk about that?" And one person said to me [when you discuss cancer and your past], "That means you're claiming in again." No what I'm claiming is complete healing, inside [and] out. From the physical point of view and from my spiritual point of view, I'm healed of that [painful memories]. I'm healed of it [breast cancer] physically. And I claim 150 percent healed of it, you know. And I plan to use this testimony over and over, until he gives me another one, you know.

While undergoing radiation, Krystal sought answers for why she had breast cancer. She searched inward. Her search led her to unresolved pains from her past. What it also led her to were realizations about God's intervention in her life. As she witnessed God working in her cancer experience, what she saw became her cancer testimony.

For Krystal, breast cancer helps her identify with other women. She uses her testimony to speak to emotional challenges women face. Her cancer testimony supports others' well-being by encouraging others to move toward self-discovery and well-being. Her testimony also supports her well-being by continually reaffirming that God has healed her, both physically and emotionally. It is her way of publically praising God. When Krystal testifies it strengthens her faith.

While some might feel uncomfortable sharing painful memories or their status as a breast cancer survivor or their past, Krystal is not ashamed. Her testimony affirms that she has been healed. Testifying is now part of Krystal's ongoing wellness.

> Everyday [I'm] getting stronger. Just whatever comes up, comes up [as a testimony]. And that's the way I am. So therefore, it doesn't rest [emotional pain]. I'm getting that stuff out. Either I pray through it or I speak through it. One way or another, I'm releasing it. So I can move on and be a source of inspiration for somebody else.

Through her testimony, Krystal continually deals with whatever emotional pain she faces. Testifying helps her release the pain. Testifying also helps her to help others. When Krystal testifies about breast cancer and her life, she inspires others' healing. Breast cancer created the platform for her testimony and opportunities to help others.

> It's [breast cancer] an avenue opened up. I think that it is part of the wellness of women. That is my major ministry—the wellness of women, the entire well-being, spiritually and physically. Now God's tying [through breast cancer] the physical in with it [her ministry and leadership]. I never looked at it this way [before cancer]. But that's [focusing on spiritual and physical well-being] a way of making the person whole.

CARLICE HARRIS—TESTIFYING FOR A PURPOSE

Carlice Harris is a retired educator and breast cancer survivor.[11] In her sixties when she was diagnosed and treated, Carlice became active in the cancer community following her diagnosis. She focuses much of her advocacy work on ensuring access to cancer information, screening, and treatment of poor women of color in urban areas. She believes wholeheartedly that these women should have access to quality care and resources just like more affluent women. Her advocacy work has led to her service on several community boards. She sees her presence as vital to influencing policies that can ultimately benefit the women and communities she represents.

When Carlice gives her cancer testimony she stands in the gap for many breast cancer survivors. Carlice believes that if nothing else, breast cancer has empowered her to speak up and to speak out. She testifies because she knows many African American breast cancer survivors feel uncomfortable doing so. Their concerns are not without merit. For in fact, testifying takes particular courage, especially for breast cancer survivors. While breast cancer survivors are often publicly praised when they reveal their cancer status, they also know that it is the equivalent of having a bull's eye on their chests. When they testify, everyone knows they have been touched by cancer.

Now, while breast cancer is less stigmatized than it has been in the past, stigma associated with breast cancer has not completely gone away. Many breast cancer survivors know this, so they choose not to divulge their cancer status. As Carlice shares,

> There are many women who do not share. And you would not know that they were survivors, unless you were close to them. They don't share and for various reasons. Sometimes people feel like you have had something when you have had cancer. [Some survivors think] that maybe they might not want to be around you for some reason or other. There are so many myths. You know like I may get it. Maybe I'll get it if I'm around her or something. There are so many reasons as to why people are afraid to tell somebody that they had it [cancer]. I think the main thing that comes to mind as to why they [survivors] don't want to be open about it is fear sometimes. And I also believe that it is [fear of] rejection because people have been rejected because they had it. And also, sometimes even, they think that somebody's going to feel sorry for me. Or they're going to think that I still do have it that I am not really healed.

> It's like once you've got it, you've always got it [cancer]. And they don't see you as being healed. They see you as, "Hey, she's got cancer."

Breast cancer survivors who choose not to reveal their cancer status do so for many reasons, including fear of rejection and other associated stigmas. Being diagnosed with breast cancer is a sensitive matter. Therefore survivors who choose not to divulge their survivorship status should be respected for the choice they make. Those that do share publicly their cancer stories are courageous because they do not know how others will perceive their cancer testimonies. Testifying, while therapeutic for some cancer survivors, is also a risky endeavor.

Carlice believes taking the risk to share her cancer testimony is worth it, no matter what others think about her. For Carlice, silence about breast cancer will not keep you from having breast cancer, so she chooses to take the risk,

> When you really learn and understand about it [cancer survivorship], you know you'd say, "Well, I don't care [what others think]. Just too bad. Tough." You look at it like you do a lot of other risks you take. You take risks all the time in your life. And you say, "Well, I'm going to do it. I can't help it. If it turns out this way, I'll accept it. If it turns out the way I want it to, I'll be happy. I'm going to take the risk."

Carlice is clear on why she is willing to take the risk. Like many cancer survivors, she initially had fears about divulging her cancer status. However, what changed her mind about sharing her cancer testimony was a change in her perspective about life and death. As Carlice says, "When you are no longer afraid to die, that is when you start living." No longer fearing death, including social death as a consequence of being stigmatized, gives Carlice the courage to share her cancer testimony.

While Carlice chooses to take the risk, other African American breast cancer survivors choose otherwise. Survivors' fears about others' response prevents many from sharing. Therefore, rather than sharing their cancer testimonies, they keep them to themselves. They mask this part of their identity from the world. For African American breast cancer survivors who already face the real social threats of racism, sexism, and elitism, not sharing one's cancer testimony serves to protect them from social fallout that might happen once their breast cancer status is known publicly.

Even though testifying publicly about breast cancer comes with the risk of being stigmatized, testifying has its own rewards. One of these rewards for Carlice is the benefit of a new perspective about breast cancer. Although Carlice views breast cancer as being a devastating disease, one that can lead to death, testifying has helped Carlice change her perspective. There are health challenges that are far worse than breast cancer she believes. When she says this during public testimonies about breast cancer, people are usually surprised. Nevertheless, she truly believes this. As she says,

> I have told people that it [breast cancer] is really not as bad as diabetes. Now I had to come to that [over a period of time]. I didn't wake up from surgery thinking that.
>
> But, coming into contact with people who [have diabetes] I say, "We [breast cancer survivors] can eat anything we want to eat. We don't have to take a shot every morning." Once we get on the road [to survivorship]. [Everything improves] once we get through with our treatment and we begin to get on the road and get back to our normal activities, which is important. I say, "It's not as bad as diabetes because once we get cured nobody tells us, 'From now on, you can't eat this anymore. You must take a shot every morning, before you eat. You must stick yourself and get some blood and check your blood sugar every morning.'"
>
> "It's not as bad," I tell them, "as emphysema." I say, "We're not struggling for every breath. We don't have to carry a breathing machine with us."

Testifying about breast cancer gives Carlice helpful perspective about the illness. There are conditions Carlice believes that are worse than breast cancer. Carlice thinks they are worse because they permanently change what people can and cannot do. This perspective helps Carlice not to let breast cancer keep her from enjoying life.

What also helps Carlice when she shares her cancer testimony is the realization that breast cancer is not something she thinks about every day. She is not bound by breast cancer. She lives life fully because she is healed. That is what she particularly likes to tell people when she testifies. As she says,

> We are not as bad off as a whole lot of other diseases like diabetes, emphysema, and probably any number of others—where you've got to get up and think about that every day. I don't think about cancer. In fact, I'm healed. So I don't have to [think about] it anymore. But, some diseases you have always got to be doing something about every day of your life. So I tell people, "It's not the worst thing that you could have." We have a tendency to think it's the worst thing you can have. But, it's not the worst thing that you can have. And when you get to live a long and active life after your diagnosis and treatment, you get cured. You go on.

Breast cancer is not the end for Carlice. It is an experience that has given her perspective about life. But, it is not stopping her. She is moving on past breast cancer. Her cancer testimony only reinforces what she believes. Breast cancer has become part of an ever-growing web of significance she has woven for her life.

Breast cancer survivors who share their cancer testimonies do so for lots of reasons. Krystal Young's and Carlice Harris's testimonies attest to this.

Some share because they do not want to bear the burden of cancer by themselves. Sharing allows others to offer them support and encouragement where needed. Cancer testimonies also affirm what they believe about themselves, namely that they have survived breast cancer. Cancer testimonies aid breast cancer survivors' personal well-being. African American breast cancer survivors' testimonies though are more than just for their benefit. These survivors' cancer testimonies also help others.

When breast cancer survivors testify publicly, they create space for others who might otherwise be reluctant to share challenges they face. People find points of commonality between their lives and those of cancer survivors. Cancer survivors' testifying creates supportive community for truth telling and healing to occur, both of which are necessary for well-being. Cancer testimonies promote well-being by attesting that change is possible. Challenges in life are not end points for these breast cancer survivors; they can be starting points for new ways of thinking and living.

As Krystal Young's and Carlice Harris's examples also suggest, testifying fosters African American cancer survivors' empowerment. It takes courage to give one's testimony about breast cancer. But these women and other African American breast cancer survivors like them do it. They do it because as the poet Audrey Lorde, who died from breast cancer said, "When we dare to be powerful, to use my strength in the service of my vision, then it becomes less and less important whether I am afraid." African American breast cancer survivors dare to be powerful by using their cancer testimonies to heal themselves and others. They also dare to use testifying, like a strategy used in the Black Church, to talk about their challenges and triumphs with breast cancer. They testify not as victims, but as overcomers. These are some of the particularly powerful aspects of African American survivors' cancer testimonies. They speak out of the depths of themselves—who they were, are, and hope to be—in service to well-being.

NOTES

1. Gilkes, C. (1993). "Womanist Ways of Seeing." In J. Cone and G. Wilmore (Eds.), *Black Theology: A Documentary History*, vol. 2, *1980–1992*, 321–324. Maryknoll, NY: Orbis Books; and Gilkes, C. (2001). *If It Wasn't for the Women. Black Women's Expeiences and Womanist Culture in Church and Community.* Maryknoll, NY: Orbis Books.
2. Lorde, A. (1980). *The Cancer Journals.* Argyle, NY: Spinsters Ink.
3. Moore, R. (2001). "African American Women and Breast Cancer: Notes from a Study of Narrative." *Cancer Nursing*, 35–43; Dunnavant, S. (1995). *Celebrating Life: African American Women Speak Out about Breast Cancer.* Dallas: USFI; and Epps, J. (1994). "On Cancer and Conjuring." In E. White (Ed.), *The Black Women's Health Book: Speaking for Ourselves*, 38–43. Seattle: Seal Press.
4. Geertz, C. (1983). *Local Knowledge: Further Essays in Interpretive Anthropology.* New York: Basic Books.
5. Ibid., 5.

6. Moore, M. (2005). "'Testifying' and 'Testimony': Autobiographcal Narratives and African American Religions." In C. Jones, and T. L. Trist (Eds.), *Teaching African American Religions*, 95–108. Oxford: Oxford University Press.

7. Ibid., 95.

8. Kleinman, A. (1988). *The Illness Narratives: Suffering, Healing and The Human Condition.* New York: Basic Books.

9. Charon, R. (2006). *Narrative Medicine: Honoring the Stories of Illness.* Oxford: Oxford University Press.

10. Krystal Young is a pseudonym and personal details of her life have been fictionalized.

11. Carlice Harris is a pseudonym and personal details of her life have been fictionalized.

Chapter Three

Black Women's Cancer Support Seeking

Black women do not experience breast cancer inside a social vacuum. Instead how Black women are perceived, how Black families and communities are perceived, and the breast cancer culture around them all influence how they respond to the disease. Each affects who African American women seek support from, how they seek support, and why they seek the types of psychosocial support they most often do. One of the most integral factors influencing how Black women with breast cancer seek social support is the "Strong Black Woman" archetype.[1]

The Strong Black Woman schema is a cultural symbol of Black womanhood and femininity that affects how others perceive Black women. This archetype also affects Black women's self-perceptions of the limits of their emotional vulnerability. Historically used as a justification and rationalization for the economic and physical exploitation of Black women during slavery,[2] the Strong Black Woman archetype presents African American women to the world as inherently strong, resilient, and self-reliant. Seemingly impervious to pain, the Strong Black Woman archetype constructs Black women as perpetually able to overcome adversity and always able to encourage others and themselves in the face of challenges. As a part of this schema, Black women's reliance on faith is often proffered as an explanation for the source of Black women's strength and self-reliance.[3] Black women are strong because God and something they are divinely endowed with makes them strong.

Consequently, Black women viewed through the lens of the Strong Black Woman archetype are characterized as stoic, resilient, and self-reliant therefore leaving little room for actual Black women with breast cancer to ask for help from others when they are in need. Their presumed ability to "go it alone" in the face of challenges reinforces Black women's silence and social isolation because to show signs of weakness or vulnerability is to risk being perceived of as "less than a woman" by one's family, peers, and the larger society. Consequently, Black women self-regulate their behavior and communicative styles in order to conform to the model of a Strong Black Woman, at times even expecting themselves to always be capable of performing this role.[4]

Black women's strong reliance on God and God talk as components of the Strong Black Woman schema can further add to their silence—particularly if they subscribe to an unexamined theology reinforced by hetero-patriarchal norms in the Black church, which emphasizes silent suffering as redemptive.[5] Black women who endure suffering by/for others to their own detriment are revered for modeling Jesus's martyrdom. Thus, to be "more like Jesus," Black women have to the kenotic, able to endure pain and ever pouring themselves out for others. Wood characterizes Black women (as a social class) who endure suffering in silence in order to maintain the socially accepted appearance of strength as "permissible victims," those who can be harmed with little or no consequence to those who hurt or perpetrate violence against them.[6]

Further adding to Black women's maintenance of the Strong Black Woman personal is the extent to which Black women, as many Black religious communities do, believe in the concept of *nommo*, which is the generative power of the spoken word.[7] Freely talking about negative situations or emotions is believed to bring about additional negative outcomes by giving verbal energy to negative situations.[8] Therefore to talk about pain, violence, or anger for some Black women with breast cancer is the equivalent of guaranteeing more pain, violence, and anger to come. As a result, Black women who model the Strong Black Woman character stifle negative emotions in order to deny them energy to further manifest, consequently making themselves more like Jesus. In a society in which African American women are rarely valued for their moral virtue or integrity, the Strong Black Woman schema, including suffering in silence and being Christ-like, becomes a double-edged sword for Black women.

To uphold the Strong Black Woman ideal requires dissemblance and suffering in silence in order to be perceived as strong. Refusing to be a Strong Black Woman by being emotionally transparent comes with the risks of being perceived as mentally weak or spiritually weak in one's faith in God and/or to be potentially exploited because of one's presumed weaknesses. Caught in the double binds of racism and sexism imbedded in the Strong Black Woman schema, Black women more often choose to internalize their pain, thereby maintaining the appearance of strength. Maintaining the appearance of outer strength while experiencing inner turmoil puts Black women at increased risk for stress-related health disparities, depression, and other negative health and mental health outcomes.[9]

Further affecting how Black women with breast cancer seek psychosocial support is the influence of the breast cancer culture itself. Sulik describes the breast cancer culture as a "set of activities, attitudes, and values that surround and shape breast cancer in public, which values selflessness, cheerfulness, unity, and optimism. A woman who is diagnosed early maintains a pleasant public and personal appearance, is optimistic, aggressively fights breast cancer, is compliant with mainstream medical advice, is an educated medical consumer, is always brave, is always victorious, and never dies."[10] The breast cancer culture perpetuates an ideal image of women with breast cancer as never sad, angry, or despondent about what happens to their bodies as a consequence of cancer treatment or uncertain about their cancer survivorship.

Added to this is the image of the "fashioned survivor," which further represents the ideal breast cancer survivor. This ideal breast cancer survivor is usually white, heterosexual, middle class, and thin.[11] As Gatison points out, what this normalization of a fashioned survivor in the context of the breast cancer culture does for Black women with breast cancer is that it alienates them from their experience and encourages silence about what hurts them, affecting how they communicate with others about their experiences. In particular, the Strong Black Woman schema, breast cancer culture, and the fashioned survivor motifs "reinforce an existing code of silence among Black women—a code that says not to talk about cancer to anyone, friend or foe."[12] Among Black women, this code , which Hine refers to as the "culture of dissemblance,"[13] makes it especially challenging for Black women to express—even with their immediate family members and friends—their feelings either about being Black women or the difficulties of experiencing breast cancer. When Black women do choose to seek support from others in coping with breast cancer they do so with many of these concerns in mind.

Despite the inherent challenges affecting their support seeking, African American breast survivors do however seek support. Their primary psychosocial buffers against cancer come from their support networks, which usually include friends and family. Black women reach for and lean on these people to cope with breast cancer. These social support networks are usually stable enough to keep survivors psychically whole. In general these networks are also pliable enough to withstand the onslaught of unique challenges Black breast cancer survivors face.

When Black breast cancer survivors are asked about what sustains their well-being during cancer, more often than not they mention family and friends. Families influence survivors' treatment decisions and support adjustments brought on by breast cancer treatment. Despite all of the benefits survivors derive from kin, at times families are ill equipped to handle some of the specific challenges these women face during cancer treatment and long-term cancer management. Families' inability to provide all of the emotional supports African American breast cancer survivors need is a fact many survivors will readily acknowledge among themselves, but not necessarily to their families or others outside of their communities. Family support, although vital to cancer recovery and survivors' well-being, has its limits.

Family members' emotional dependency on survivors makes it difficult for some to be sensitive to survivors' needs. Family members do care. Yet, competing priorities make providing consistent support a challenge. Family members often live in the same house and share the same resources (i.e., space, money, etc.) with the survivor. Family members also often expect survivors to function to their fullest capacities as spouses, mothers, providers, and caretakers. Survivors are generally expected to suspend their sick role functioning and resume the roles they assumed prior to diagnosis and treatment.[14] Some survivors, however, as a consequence of cancer treatment, are unable to resume their pre-diagnosis functioning, either for an extended period of time and/or indefinitely. As a result, family members' focus can shift away from what survivors feel or may express about their physical or emotional health.

Although families are important to survivors' coping, families are at times simply ill-equipped to provide the emotional support necessary for Black women with breast cancer. Rather than risk their families being perceived as weak because of their inability to support Black cancer survivors throughout their breast cancer experience, some Black women choose to keep critiques of family members' support to themselves. Black women make do with what they receive from their families and do not complain about what is lacking in the familial support their receive.

When survivors need more than their families' emotional resources can provide, they seek support from friends and others (e.g., clergy, other cancer survivors, health-care professionals). Supportive others have greater social distance from survivors' immediate disease/illness situations. Friends often empathize or sympathize in ways that demonstrate to survivors that somebody really hears them. Friends listen and understand without needing every detail of what survivors experience explained. Friends express through the support they provide that African American survivors' need for support is not a personal failing. Instead, supportive others convey that support, both its provision and receipt, which is essential for well-being. Friendship is enmeshed with certain expectations about providing mutual support, which makes it particularly helpful to Black women survivors' coping.

Black survivors seek social support from friends, family, and supportive others in culturally patterned ways. These women's intersectional identities of race, class, and gender particularly influence how they seek support. Their social identities and histories suggest why African American breast cancer survivors' support seeking is important for well-being. Black breast cancer survivors need support because too often they mask their feelings of distress (i.e., dissemblance). With few outlets for support, African American women historically have used their reciprocal support relationships with each other as friends to meet their material and emotional needs. Through kin, friendships, and other supportive relationships, Black women provided social support for each other in African American communities.

Historically, activation of these African American women's support networks, usually in racially segregated communities, led to organized efforts like the establishment of schools, hospitals, banks, along with various social, political, and religious organizations.[15] Reciprocal support sharing among Black women has been characterized as "making community" or social mobilization to organize and institute efforts needed to support African American survival.[16] In many African American women's early efforts in the twentieth century, to share social support, Black women functioned as "race women" whose explicit interests and agency focused to achieve social, political, and economic well-being for African American communities. Black women providing social support to each other was not just interpersonal sharing, but also sharing for community development and uplift.

Contemporary Black women continue to evidence community making in their social support seeking and mutual aid efforts in relation to breast cancer.[17] Mutual aid, as an intentional set of behaviors from which formalized mutual aid societies and efforts like schools and organizations often result, is purposeful. Intended to support adaptation to new and dynamic social situations, mutual aid supports African Americans' coping and psychosocial adjustment. Mutual aid is often initiated to alleviate pain and suffering associated with sickness and death,[18] thus it is outcome driven. African American cancer survivors' support seeking in relation to breast cancer does both. It supports Black survivors' coping by alleviating their emotional pain and suffering, which improves their well-being.

Black breast cancer survivors purposefully seek and give mutual aid to each other as part of their cancer experiences. They do this to cope and adapt to changes cancer brings to the social, economic, emotional, and physical landscape of their lives. Black cancer survivors experience complex life changes, therefore their attempts at support seeking are not haphazard. African American breast cancer survivors' mutual aid seeking is culturally patterned and logical. They seek support from people they trust, those they can racially identify with and culturally relate to, and from those they believe have their best interests in mind and will not use their emotional vulnerability against them. Black women with cancer also seek support from those who do not confine them to adhering to the dictates of the breast cancer culture, fashioned survivor, or Strong Black Woman schemas. This often means that when Black breast cancer survivors seek support outside of their families, they do so with people they are racially concordant with, who understand Black culture, or who are familiar with breast cancer treatment and its long-term effects.

In this study, mutual aid specifically refers to psychosocial support African American breast cancer survivors seek from people other than family members. Mutual aid for these cancer survivors serves several cultural functions. It is the behavioral strategy Black breast cancer survivors use to acquire social support. It encompasses the people, places, and situations where social support is received. Mutual aid also manifests as a by-product of African American cancer survivors' support seeking. It includes the informational, social, and emotional supports Black breast cancer survivors provide to others. African American breast cancer survivors seeking and receiving mutual aid, as well as giving mutual aid, support their total well-being.

Beyond their families, Black breast cancer survivors often talk about reliance on faith communities (i.e., churches), church members, friends, and clergy (i.e., ministers) for social support. Survivors receive support from their mutual aid networks in socially acceptable ways, usually in keeping with their cultural and religious beliefs (i.e., testifying about experiences, communality, etc.). Black breast cancer survivors also use these mutual aid networks to offer ideas and support to benefit others' well-being, therefore serving as sources of encouragement for others.

Through African American breast cancer survivors' mutual aid use, they typically generate and foster an oppositional consciousness about breast cancer. Instead of focusing on the increased likelihood of dying from breast cancer because they are Black, female, or have high-risk cancer types, the Black cancer survivors' mutual aid networks in this study promote an oppositional consciousness that stresses survival against the prevailing odds. This oppositional consciousness does not discount the realities of Black women's higher mortality when diagnosed or poorer long-term survival rates. Instead, this oppositional consciousness fashions Black survivors' hopes into a visionary pragmatism that disease-free / illness-free survival is possible for them because engaging principally with other Black women surviving breast cancer reinforces this possibility.

In other mutual aid contexts (e.g., ministerial counseling), Black breast cancer survivors benefit from and help others. Survivors' abilities to give and receive support reflect their moral ethics regarding charity and benevolence and demonstrate their belief in a womanist spirituality of survival.[19] African American cancer survivors believe they can do something to affect their survival. This spirituality of survival evidenced as survivors' traditional communalism[20] compels them to nurture and support others out of love for God and others. When Black cancer survivors share their knowledge and resources they do so for others' well-being and their own.

Outside of religious/spiritual contexts, African American breast cancer survivors also seek mutual aid within their broader social networks. Support comes from friends and others—especially those who particularly understand breast cancer (e.g., other Black cancer survivors, health-care professionals). Black breast cancer survivors find in these supportive others additional ways to think about and cope with breast cancer. Opportunities to exchange social support in these mutual aid contexts give African American breast cancer survivors additional information and perspective to inform their coping. Black breast cancer survivors often find these mutual aid experiences to be gratifying, particularly when they are not required to perform as Strong Black women or in accordance to the dominant breast cancer culture.

Although on the whole Black breast cancer survivors find support seeking in the context of mutual aid to be emotionally satisfying, sometimes their support-seeking efforts fall short in meeting the expected quality of mutual aid delivery and/or providing the outcomes they expected. When this happens, some Black cancer survivors use their negative experiences with support seeking to refine their future support seeking and to evaluate the quality of other social support they receive. Black cancer survivors' use of mutual aid in these specific ways evidences at least four cultural functions for African American breast cancer survivors.

Mutual aid for Black cancer survivors functions as a support-seeking and support-provision behavioral strategy. When social support is sought, it is sought as a psychosocial output, which minimizes emotional distress by restoring psychosocial balance. Mutual aid further functions as an evaluative tool Black women use to gauge the quality and effectiveness of all social support they receive. Lastly, mutual aid serves as a catalyzing force, which influences Black breast cancer survivors' future behaviors to promote their well-being. Williams and Williams have described these first two cultural functions of mutual aid historically among African Americans.[21] The latter two are unique to this study.

As a case study, one African American cancer survivor's experience is described. It serves as the basis for making theoretical claims about African American breast cancer survivors' mutual aid seeking. Evidenced in this survivor's story are concerns about breast cancer culture, the fashioned survivor image, and the Strong Black Woman schema and how these led to her conflicted feelings about what she considered to be socially inappropriate emotions. How these competing concerns also affected her support-seeking behaviors is also evident. The meanings this survivor gives to her mutual aid experiences and how these relate to other Black breast cancer survivors' coping abilities will also further be considered.

TRACY SPARKS—HOLDING ON TO MUTUAL AID

Tracy Sparks, a fifty-two-year-old single mother, works for a social service agency.[22] Tracy was diagnosed with breast cancer on two occasions. Since her last recurrence, Tracey is now a four-year breast cancer survivor. Diagnosed initially at the age of twenty-nine, Tracy underwent a radical mastectomy, followed by chemotherapy. With her recurrence at the age of forty-seven, Tracy had another mastectomy. With the first cancer diagnosis, Tracy felt shock and fear. With her cancer recurrence she felt anger, with God and herself. Tracey's anger however was not readily apparent to her at the time of her second diagnosis.

Despite how she felt, Tracy was raised to believe that anger was not an emotion Black women should express. Therefore, when Tracey felt angry she experienced tremendous emotional turmoil because she had few socially sanctioned outlets for its expression. She considered emotional outbursts and visible outrage, particularly as a Black woman in the South, to be unacceptable. As a result, Tracey turned her anger and other emotional distress inward following her breast cancer diagnoses. Tracy says she learned to effectively mask her pain behind food and binge eating. Research suggests that binge eating is a common maladaptive behavior many Black women who internalize the Strong Black Woman schema use to avoid, distract from, or escape trauma reminders Black women experience.[23] Tracy used overeating to soothe her pain and dissemble.

Displaying an outwardly jovial nature was another way Tracy dissembled her true feelings. Tracy became particularly adept at keeping her feelings hidden following her first cancer diagnosis. She became even more adroit at emotionally masking after her cancer recurrence.

Despite her best efforts, Tracy's pain and anger resulting from breast cancer refused to be ignored. These emotions continued to bubble to the surface in her thoughts and actions. As Tracy explains, she needed to find ways to process what she was feeling inside. Seeking support through mutual aid became a behavioral strategy she used to help her do this. Tracy looked for and found mutual aid through various outlets, including other survivors, her physicians, ministerial counseling, as well as organized groups. Each mutual aid experience helped Tracy reconnect with the bottled up emotions she kept inside. Her mutual aid encounters moved Tracy closer toward her desired outcome—emotional and psychosocial recovery and well-being. Achieving these outcomes were a process for Tracy.

Tracy reflects on feelings she had subsequent to her recurrence. She remembers feeling this way:

> I was just real angry. For a while even my faith [in God] just wasn't there. Just wasn't there. Even afterward, they told me, "Yes, they caught it in the zero to

> less than one percent range" and that because of that I didn't have to have chemotherapy. That was good, but I still couldn't get over that [recurrence]. It was like the fear that I'm going through this all over again. And just for a while I was real angry. It took me a while to work through that anger before I could accept that it was okay. But, I felt hurt that God had allowed this to happen.

Tracy recalls feeling several simultaneous emotions with her cancer recurrence. She was angry with God about having breast cancer after her initial diagnosis. Her anger only grew following her recurrence. Although both cancers had been detected and treated in their early stages, Tracy was afraid and felt as if God had betrayed her twice by allowing her to be diagnosed on two separate occasions.

Masking her pain and anger, Tracy maintained her usual routines and social roles. She kept working, taking care of her daughter, and participating in other social activities. On the outside, it appeared that Tracy was coping well with cancer. But, the real emotions she felt remained bottled up inside. Tracy needed support, but she had not found the type of support she particularly needed. She found this needed support several years later. She remembers one of her first encounters with a supportive relationship, indicative of mutual aid,

> I only talked [at first, after my initial diagnosis] with one other person. And that had been through my meeting with Tiffany. And I didn't meet her until [twelve years after my initial diagnosis]. Not too long after I started at Cooper's [the company I work for]. We just started talking and it was just good to have somebody to talk to and process it [my feelings]. And share. She would share with me her feelings and I would share with her.
>
> [I had not sought support beyond this friendship because] I guess at this point it would have been the amount of time that had passed since I was initially diagnosed. That would be one reason. The other reason [for not seeking organized support] would be not having [access to] a group with African American women. I mean I would have been more comfortable [with such a group], even though I went to a group at the "Y" [YWCA] right after my surgery. I went to that although it fizzled out. But, I really would have enjoyed the experience of going through that [the breast cancer experience] with other African American women.

Tracy found her friendship with another African American breast cancer survivor to be emotionally beneficial, even twelve years after her initial diagnosis. Although Tracy sought support from an organized group after her initial surgery, it did not fully address her needs. Tracy wanted social support from other Black cancer survivors. Tracy's desire for social support from people she shared racial concordance with reflects her overall orientation to health-care seeking.

Health-care coverage policies and health-maintenance organization restrictions limit Tracy's abilities to seek medical care exclusively from African American physicians. She prefers having Black health-care providers treating her. This is a preference she has held throughout her life. Tracy's parents raised her to believe that African American health-care providers, by virtue of their shared ethnicity and culture, will be more sensitive to the needs and concerns of African American patients. Tracy remembers her parents' lesson this way:

> The message from my parents was "Get you a Black doctor." I mean they were very, very strong messages. "Get you a Black doctor because they will take care of you. They'll be fair with you and they'll treat you with respect."

Tracy's experiences with African American physicians lived up to her expectations. African Americans' history of negative encounters with biomedicine in the United States further substantiated Tracy's confidence in Black health-care professionals. For her, it is both rational and culturally appropriate to seek support and care from Black health-care providers because presumably these people will not exploit or mistreat their Black patients. When a Black doctor is not available, Tracy uses the next best alternative.

In seeking social support, Tracy sought out mutual aid through a local and well-established social service agency in her community. She felt comfortable seeking mutual aid from this organization because its mission aligned with her faith orientation. Tracy used this group's mutual aid until the group disbanded. She continued to use this group for support even though, as she admits, it did not fully provide the type of support she wanted.

After this first experience with organized mutual aid, Tracy decided not to seek additional social support—that is, until she started a friendship with another African American cancer survivor, named Tiffany Jones.[24] In Tracy's friendship with Tiffany she found social support that met her needs and reflected the type of racially concordant support she wanted. Although attending the organized support group helped some and her friendship with Tiffany was also beneficial, Tracy sought other support encounters to benefit her well-being. For Tracy, her oncologist became another supportive person in her mutual aid network. Tracy talks about her encounter with her oncologist this way:

> [I also used another kind of support] It is kind of informal. My oncologist used to listen to me. And he was just real supportive and gave me feedback. He would give me supportive feedback when I needed it. But the main thing was he listened to me. That Jewish doctor had nothing in common with me. He was a man, a Jewish doctor, and young. By him doing that and listening to me, it made the chemotherapy not such a bad experience. The chemo itself was a real

bad experience. But I would leave him, go to my chemotherapy, and it was like I was just kind of calm. And it was okay.

As a result of Tracy's lack of faith in health-care providers who are not African American, she was particularly surprised by the social support she received from her oncologist. In Tracy's estimation, she and her oncologist shared little in common. However, what they did share was a mutual commitment to Tracy's receiving the best cancer care possible. This shared commitment to Tracy's well-being was sufficient to establish a trusting relationship between Tracy and her oncologist. Even though he was young, male, and Jewish, Tracy's oncologist cared enough about her well-being to actively listen to her concerns about chemotherapy and cancer. Tracy did not fear that expressing her vulnerability with her oncologist would later be used against her.

Tracy dreaded chemotherapy and she became increasingly more anxious with each round she had. However Tracy's oncologist's receptive and supportive demeanor allayed much of her anxiety and made chemotherapy less distressing. Tracy's oncologist became part of her widening mutual aid network of support. This was precipitated by the fact that her oncologist did not expect Tracy to conform to any particular model of how a breast cancer patient should respond to treatment. Instead of self-monitoring her behavior, Tracy was free to be herself, including being emotionally vulnerable and transparent with her feelings about chemotherapy.

When Tracy was initially diagnosed with breast cancer she turned to others for social support. She turned notably to a minister. Tracy describes the benefits she received while going through chemotherapy to treat her initial cancer.

> I talked to a minister during that time. And even afterward, even up to four years afterward [her initial diagnosis], I talked to a minister about my experience. It was something I initiated. I needed to talk to someone. Some things were coming up and I was able to process it with a minister. It was good. It was good. He, of course being male, he didn't know about breast cancer. But he was able to listen and help me work through my feelings. [I used this counseling initially] for about four months. This was after treatment [for my initial cancer].

The social support Tracy received from this minister was different from her other supportive encounters she had. Tracy used these sessions with this minister to process her feelings. Although he was male and had never had breast cancer, his professional role provided the skills needed to help Tracy work through her feelings. The emotional clarity she received during these exchanges supported her well-being process. Of note is that this minister was not a part of the breast cancer culture, therefore he was not wedded to an image of how Tracy as a breast cancer survivor should act. Consequently, his willingness to allow Tracy to express her true feelings without the added work of self-regulating her feelings provided the opportunities needed for her to genuinely express what she felt.

Mutual aid offered through additional friendships and spiritual fellowships also provided Tracy with needed social support. As she shares,

> A prayer group [also helped me cope.] A year afterward [after the initial diagnosis] I went to this little church with one of my co-workers at Cooper's [where I worked]. And every Wednesday night I would go. And it was just a little group. And it was just a little rinky-dink church. But, it was just something that at that time fed my spiritual needs. That helped me at that particular time.

African American breast cancer survivors' mutual aid networks are often eclectic and the social supports they receive are equally varied. The church prayer group Tracy attended weekly did not provide individualized counseling, case management, or other supportive cancer survivorship services that perhaps would have been helpful to Tracy. Despite the group's seeming limitations, Tracy found sufficient social support to benefit her spiritual well-being.

The Wednesday night prayer group in this predominantly Black church similar was beneficial for reasons similar to what she received from her oncologist, ministerial counseling, and other mutual aid encounters. This group did not require Tracy to adhere to a predetermined model of either a breast cancer survivor or Strong Black Woman. Here, Tracy could be genuine with a group of people who, just like her, faced life challenges. What they did not share in experience they made up for in shared belief that prayer, talking, and seeking support from God by gathering collectively could resolve the issues they had. Their shared relief seeking from suffering and pain, indicative of mutual aid, made this group and what it offered of greatest benefit to Tracy. Surrounded by people who did not think less of her for being weak, because they too were weak and in need, made Tracy feel better because she knew she was not alone.

Tracy, like many African American breast cancer survivors, used her social support seeking and encounters with those in her mutual aid network in a triangulated fashion. From each encounter she acquired information and behavioral strategies supportive to her well-being. As her network broadened and her experiences varied, Tracy became better equipped to deal with emotions breast cancer produced for her. Her mutual aid network lessened her suffering and distress. It did this specifically by giving Tracy coping strategies she consciously applied to identify and work through challenging emotions she felt. As Tracy applied these strategies, she also used encounters with those in her mutual aid network to evaluate her coping and continually assess her well-being.

Tracy's use of mutual aid as a type of emotional feedback loop is sophisticated. Seeking and receiving social support benefits her ongoing well-being. As Tracy shares,

> I used to have a real hard time working through feelings and expressing my feelings. Not only expressing them to others, but to myself. It takes me a while to just process, to just get in touch with what it is that I'm feeling. In these support [situations] they helped me first get in touch with my feelings. I'm sometimes so good at masking [my feelings] that sometimes I knew that something just didn't feel right on the inside. But, as I was allowed a space and the environment to talk, I could get in touch with "Yeah, this is what it is."
>
> And even if I wasn't able to identify it at the time, it provided [a way for me to go back] later. I might have said, "Okay. This is what this is. And this is why I'm feeling it." I could go back and take it back to the group. And they would listen and I could get it out. And [these mutual aid situations] have ways of dealing with whatever the feeling was.
>
> See, part of the support—even the prayer group, the one I went to for almost a year and then it dissolved after I became a parent—had therapists in them [as participants]. And so we all had a format to heal thyself and to work through the process. That was the process of identifying, talking about the feeling, and learning how to deal with it in healthy ways.

As an emotional feedback loop, Tracy describes how encounters with people in her mutual aid network helped her to immediately identify with the feelings she had. These encounters and the process of dealing with emotions they provided also became reference points for Tracy during later reflection periods.

For African American breast cancer survivors, support found in mutual aid encounters and social networks are particularly helpful in dealing with emotions these cancer survivors find difficult to deal with otherwise. Tracy had a particularly difficult time processing her feelings of anger. Having few outlets to talk about anger, particularly as a Black woman, Tracy kept these feelings particularly bottled up. Instead of expressing her angry feelings and working through them, Tracy, like many Black women with breast cancer, buried them. Burying her anger proved detrimental to Tracy's well-being. Nevertheless this is what Tracy did because having internalized the Strong Black Woman schema she believed this was what was expected of her. Having tried to live up to being the Strong Black Woman, one unaffected by pain or anger, Tracy came to expect this of herself. That is, until she found outlets, through her mutual aid network, to express her anger. Tracy shares,

> [This process of the prayer group helped me deal with] Anger. Anger was always one of those not okay feelings. And the biggest thing I had was I was

> just angry at God. And I didn't realize that I was angry at him for putting me through this experience. [I did not acknowledge that fact] that I had to go through all of this. But I covered it up. It wasn't until later in '95 [1995], when I went [back] to counseling with the minister [after my breast cancer recurrence], that I got in touch with that. And then I was able to work through that. [Counseling sessions with the minister gave me the opportunity] to just cry and just let it go [of anger]. And [in those sessions I] worked toward [understanding] God is a loving God. And that he has been with me through this experience.

Tracy found ministerial counseling useful because it allowed her to acknowledge feelings of anger, feelings she had not previously recognized and were contrary to what breast cancer culture identifies as socially acceptable. When Tracy identified how she felt, these supportive sessions then helped her to identify with whom she was angry. She was angry with God. This was something she had covered up, perhaps seeing this as a direct violation of what it means to be a Strong Black Woman whose faith in God is unquestioned.

When Tracy acknowledged how she felt and whom her anger was directed toward, she could work through her feelings. Instead of generating more anger toward God, talking about her anger had the opposite effect. It gave Tracy greater peace. Ministerial counseling helped Tracy reappraise her thoughts about God, especially in relation to her cancer experience. Instead of seeing God as punitive, Tracy reconsidered her ideas about God. She eventually saw God as one who was continually present in her experience with cancer. Tracy's recognition of her true feelings, release of her pent up feelings, and reappraisal of her feelings about God and theology supported her well-being.

Tracy's experience underscores that Black survivors' achievement of well-being is an ongoing process. For many survivors, achieving well-being also includes moments of theological challenge and even spiritual crisis. Wrestling with conflicted feelings about God is common. Black cancer survivors' spirituality of survival affirms God's presence in their disease/illness experience, however Black cancer survivors, even those who internalize a Strong Black Woman schema, do not always view God's presence positively.

Tracy was initially angry with God and blamed God for giving her breast cancer. Yet because of her strong identification with being a Strong Black Woman, one who suffers in silence and does not talk about negative situations, Tracy kept her feelings to herself out of concern that her feelings were not appropriate. As is typical with many African American breast cancer survivors, Tracy's reappraisal of God and amending of her theology occurred throughout her breast cancer experience. It happened in conjunction with her search for cancer's meaning in her life. As she clarified her feelings about God, Tracy thought about God differently.

Instead of being vindictive, Tracy came to view God as supportive. Because Tracy's spirituality of survival envisioned God as always present, her amended theology allowed her conflicting feelings toward God to be held in tension until she could reconcile her feelings about God. What Tracy determined was that being angry with God did not mean she or her faith in God was weak. She also discovered that repressing her feelings did not make her more virtuous in the same way her silence did not prevent her from experiencing more emotional pain. It was only when Tracy acknowledged her true feelings that she was able to reconcile her theology and find peace with herself and her pain.

A spirituality of survival, which comes out of Black women's lived theology of God, allows Black breast cancer survivors to have conflicting feelings toward God and their experiences with breast cancer. The nurturing of this spirituality of survival often happens in the context of African American cancer survivors' support-seeking behaviors and mutual aid networks. Both are particularly relevant in relation to Black women's historic masking of their true feelings to maintain the image of the Strong Black Woman. A repeated theme in Tracy's life is masking. Masking behind the image of being a Strong Black Woman had been one of Tracy's most successful coping strategies. This same coping strategy serves other Black breast cancer survivors in their personal and professional lives as well.

As an African American cultural survival strategy, masking, as part of the Strong Black Woman schema, requires Black women to sublimate their true feelings in response to actualities in their lives, particularly painful or traumatic events. Scholars of African American women's history refer to this phenomenon as a "culture of dissemblance."[25] Hines describes Black women's emotional masking as, "behavior and attitudes of black women that created the appearance of openness and disclosure but actually shielded the truth of their inner lives and selves from their oppressors."[26] Black women, particularly as a consequence of racism and sexism, learn often from their families to keep how they truly feel to themselves and instead take on the persona of the Strong Black Woman—silent in suffering, faithful to God, and self-reliant. Many Black women continue to use this strategy in response to breast cancer. Black breast cancer survivors often mask, from others and even themselves, how they truly feel.

Tracy describes how she learned to mask her feelings early in life. Her mother taught her this strategy. As Tracy shares,

> [If I have been mistreated] the majority of the time I keep it to myself. I internalize it. I accept it as a fact of life. Part of it was my training. You know the messages that I received from my parents. Just turn the others cheek and just go on. And [by doing] that you would show then that you're a bigger person against them. Just ignore them. I can remember as a kid having to go

downtown and having to go to the bathroom and the woman said we had to go to the basement in one of the department stores. I was about seven. And my mother said, "Oh no. She has to go now. So she is going to use this bathroom." And my mother was called the N-word. And then she said to me, "Just ignore it. Just ignore it. And you show them that you're a bigger person by not saying anything." And I learned to take that as a message I learned growing up.

Tracy's mother taught her how to dissemble by acting like a Strong Black Woman in order to cope with an oppressively hostile world. Tracy continues to dissemble and be a Strong Black Woman as a cultural survival strategy. She is not alone. Many Black breast cancer survivors dissemble their true feelings about having breast cancer. Because African American breast cancer survivors were often taught early in life how to be the Strong Black Woman, as adults they are almost unaware that they are doing it.

They might be angered and/or frustrated by the circumstances of breast cancer, however Black women learn to suppress how they truly feel. In place of anger or frustration, in keeping with the Strong Black Woman schema and breast cancer culture, Black women present themselves to the world as always upbeat, jovial, stoic, or resolute in response to challenges and trauma, including breast cancer. Dissemblance has been a useful tool of social engagement and psychosocial resistance historically for Black women. Nevertheless, the Strong Black Woman schema and the model of an ideal survivor from breast cancer culture have their limits. At the same time that being strong and dissembling has allowed African American women to deal with oppression, it has negative consequences.

For African American breast cancer survivors, masking and the Strong Black Woman schema are strategies for developing oppositional consciousness (e.g., fighting racism, sexism); however, they have detrimental effects on well-being. Black breast cancer survivors who regularly dissemble suffer as a consequence of it. Survivors who dissemble shield their truest emotional selves to prevent being perceived as weak. Yet, Black women like Tracy do this to an extent where they become psychologically detached from their own feelings. This happened to Tracy. Here she reflects on the negative psychological effects of dissembling. As she said,

I internalize [my feelings]. I was raised to internalize my feelings. And in my life I've learned how to deal with them in negative ways. In trying, it's a whole lot harder to break those patterns. Now I know that when I want something to eat or want something sweet, then there's something going on within me. When I can't sleep, then I know it's something that I'm not processing or I'm not in tune with. I've used this survival technique for so long that it takes me a couple of days to process.

I always say I have delayed reactions. It takes me two or three days before I get in touch with what the feeling is and what caused that feeling. Then I can

> work through it, whereas [as] I used to [be], I wouldn't. Now I have a delayed reaction to responding, but at least I respond.

Tracy learned to dissemble and to be a Strong Black Woman early in life. She became so adroit at doing it she has difficulty identifying stressful feelings she has. Overeating and outward joviality served as Tracy's primary masks for her feelings. While she used these initially in response to her cancer diagnoses, she realized these would not work long-term. Tracy's need for social support to examine her feelings and identify healthful coping strategies spurred her use of mutual aid.

Mutual aid in all of the relationships where she located it gave Tracy spaces and opportunities to unmask emotionally. Tracy could be herself. She did not have to be jovial, strong or resilient if this was not how she felt. She could be angry or frustrated and not be judged harshly for it. Tracy also found in these relationships opportunities to identify her anger with God and not feel bad for it. Tracy found in these mutual aid experiences opportunities to acknowledge her feelings, process what she had experienced, and begin to heal emotionally. None of these supportive people or spaces required her to perform as a Strong Black Woman or an ideal breast cancer survivor.

Black women diagnosed with breast cancer particularly need social support. Families provide a lot of this support. In ways families cannot, friends and supportive others are often better equipped to offer cancer survivors support they need. African American breast cancer survivors draw emotionally from friends and supportive others. These supportive relationships function as the mutual aid networks African American breast cancer survivors develop to support well-being.

African American breast cancer survivors cannot always determine when, where, or from whom they will receive social support. The social support cancer survivors seek and receive may be consistent or intermittently provided in their mutual aid networks. How long support is offered or the length of time between when cancer survivors receive support does not negate its importance in their lives. What is most important is what mutual aid does for African American breast cancer survivors. What it does at its best is alleviate Black cancer survivors' emotional suffering, allowing them to unmask and authentically be themselves. When and where Black women process their unresolved feelings and arrive at emotional healing—these are the places where their well-being happens.

NOTES

1. Beauboeuf-Lafonrant, Tamara. (2009). *Behind the Mask of the Strong Black Woman: Voice and the Embodiments of a Costly Performance.* Philadelphia: Temple University Press; and Hamilton-Mason, J., Hall, J. C., and Everette, J. E. (2009). "And Some of Us Are Braver:

Stress and Coping among African American Women." *Journal of Human Behavior in the Social Environment*: 463–482.

2. Harris-Lacewell, M. (2001). "No Place to Rest: African American Political Attitudes and the Myth of Black Women's Strength." *Women and Politics, 23*, 1–33; and Collins, Patricia Hill. (2000). *Black Feminist Thought: Knowledge, Consciousness, and the Politics of Empowerment.* New York: New York University Press.

3. Gatison, Annette. (2015). "The Pink and Black Experience: Lies that Make Us Suffer in Silence and Cost Us Our Lives." *Women's Studies in Communication, 38*, 135–140.

4. Beauboeuf-Lafontant, Tamara. (2008). "Listening Past the Lies That Make Us Sick: A Voice-Centered Analysis of Strength and Depression among Black Women." *Qualitative Sociology, 31*, 391–406.

5. Wood, Frances. (1993). "'Take My Yoke upon You': The Role of the Church in the Oppression of African-American Women." In Emilie Townes (Ed.), *A Troubling in My Soul: Womanist Perspectives On Evil & Suffering*, 37–47. Maryknoll, NY: Orbis Books.

6. Ibid., 46.

7. Jackson, R., and Richardson, E. (Eds.). (2003). *Understanding African American Rhetoric: Classical and Contemporary Innovations.* New York: Routledge.

8. Gatison, "The Pink and Black Experience," 137.

9. Parks, S. (2010). *Fierce Angels: The Strong Black Woman in American Life and Culture.* New York: Random House; Hill, S. A. (2009). "Cultural Images and the Health of African American Women." *Gender and Society, 23* (6): 733–746; and Woods-Giscombe, Cheryl. (2010). "Superwoman Schema: African American Women's Views on Stress, Strength and Health." *Qualitative Health Research, 20* (5): 668–683.

10. Sulik, G. A. (2010). *Pink Ribbon Blues: How Breast Cancer Culture Undermines Women's Health.* New York: Oxford University Press.

11. Ucok, O. (2007). "The Fashioned Survivor: Institutionalized Representations of Women with Breast Cancer." *Communication and Medicine, 4* (1): 67–78.

12. Gatison, "The Pink and Black Experience," 136.

13. Hine, Darlene. (1994). *Hine Sight: Black Women and the Re-construction of American History.* Bloomington: Indiana University Press.

14. Parsons, Talcott. (1951). *The Social System.* Glencoe, IL: Free Press.

15. Higginbotham, Elizabeth. (1993). *Righteous Discontent: The Women's Movement in the Black Church, 1880–1920.* Cambridge, MA: Harvard University Press; Brown, E. (1994). "Womanist Consciousness: Maggie Lena Walker and the Independent Order of Saint Luke." In V. Ruiz and E. DuBois (Eds.), *Unequal Sisters: A Multicultural Reader in U.S. Women's History*, 268–283. New York: Routledge; and Shaw, Stephanie. (1996). *What a Woman Ought to Be and to Do: Black Professional Women Workers during the Jim Crow Era.* Chicago: University of Chicago Press.

16. Hine. *Hine Sight*, xxii.

17. Williams, Charles, and Williams, Hilda. (1992). "Mutual Aid Societies and Economic Development: Survival Efforts." In Hans Baer and Yvonne Jones (Eds.), *African Amercians in the South: Issues of Race, Class and Gender*. Athens: University of Georgia Press.

18. Ibid., 26.

19. Brown-Douglass, K. (1993). "Womanist Theology: What Is Its Relationship to Black Theology?" In James Cone and G. Wilmore (Eds.), *Black Theology: A Documentary History*, vol. 2, *1980–1992*, 290–299. Maryknoll, NY: Orbis Books.

20. Floyd-Thomas, Stacey (Ed.). (2006). *Deeper Shades of Purple.* New York: NYU Press.

21. Williams and Williams. "Mutual Aid Societies and Economic Development."

22. Tracy Sparks is a pseudonym and personal details about her life have been fictionalized.

23. Harrington, Ellen, Crowther, Janis, and Shipherd, Julian. (2010). "Trauma, Binge Eating, and the 'Strong Black Woman.'" *Journal of Counseling and Clinical Psychology, 78* (4): 469–479.

24. Tiffany Jones is a pseudonym.

25. Hine. *Hine Sight*, 37–47.

26. Ibid., 37.

Chapter Four

Healing Claims as Acts of Faith and Resistance

High breast cancer mortality rates among African American women have been attributed to many things, including cultural beliefs.[1] While recent research indicates that many African American women experience more aggressive breast cancer types[2] and are exposed to other risk factors (i.e., poverty) and systemic barriers (i.e., poorer quality care) that comprise their outcomes,[3] ideas about African American women and fatalism following cancer diagnoses still persist. Fatalism, the inability to control one's destiny or fate or resignation in the face of death, has been suggested as a reason for why African American women delay seeking treatment for breast cancer.[4] Fatalism has also been used to explain some African American cancer survivors' medical noncompliance with recommended cancer treatment.[5] African American breast cancer survivors' presumed fatalism is often seen as connected to their faith in God.

Black breast cancer survivors who assert a strong faith in God in response to breast cancer are viewed by some in the medical community as in denial about their health or the disease's progression. Believing these survivors to be either incapable of understanding medical information or detached from reality, African American breast cancer survivors who prefer to trust in God in response to late-stage cancer diagnoses or appear unafraid about death are easily stigmatized. As a consequence, African American breast cancer survivors are easily stereotyped as fatalists and their beliefs about God are marginalized within cancer care settings, reinforcing beliefs about African Americans as a problematic or ignorant population.[6] In response, some Black breast cancer survivors, as an act of resistance, keep their thoughts about God to themselves rather than openly share what they believe (i.e., their cultural theology) with their health-care providers.

What happens as a result is that fatalism becomes a persistent explanation for African American women's actions in response to breast cancer. Not understood as part of a larger cultural theology African American cancer survivors have about how God functions, breast cancer survivors' faith in God can be easily misunderstood as a barrier to care. Challenging misunderstandings regarding African American breast cancer survivors and their medical decision-making is important to improving care, a point that has been noted.[7] Also understanding how African American breast cancer survivors' reliance on God, particularly with late-stage cancer diagnoses and in response to death, functions as acts of resistance are also important.

Key to Black cancer survivors' strong reliance on God as their locus of resistance to breast cancer is understanding how African American women conceptualize pain and suffering. The late poet Audre Lorde, who died of breast cancer, makes a distinction between pain and suffering.[8] For Lorde, suffering is pain that is neither scrutinized nor processed. It is the recurring cycle of pain that can be triggered by events or people, like ruminating on a terminal cancer diagnosis or fearing death. That kind of suffering is what leads to oppression. Pain, by contrast, is the recognized naming of one's experience for the intent of transformation.

As the womanist theologian Townes notes, Black women who subscribe to a womanist theology that rejects suffering as God's will, respond by struggling against suffering.[9] Suffering, as part of this Black women's cultural theology, is seen as sinful because it relies on self to overcome sin and injustice, instead of relying on God for deliverance. When Black women resist suffering by struggling against the sources of suffering (i.e., terminal cancer diagnosis, fears about death, racism, sexism) their trust is located in Jesus's resurrection event, which is believed to have removed true suffering, thereby redeeming believers from experiencing it. Those who are liberated from suffering use their pain as fuel for struggle. Townes asserts, "The resurrection is God's breaking into history to transform suffering into wholeness—to move the person from victim to change agent."[10] Black women who believe this way rely on faith in God to resist suffering and struggle against breast cancer's indignities. The resurrection is the locus for Black women cancer survivors' faith in healing and wholeness.

Regardless of what the cancer prognosis is, these Black women know that with God "everything will be alright." They work through their pain by acknowledging their ability to effect change in their lives. Rather than accept the "facts" of breast cancer handed to them, these cancer survivors choose to live despite the facts. Their pain allows these survivors to examine their lives and make plans for their futures. And although on the outside their strong reliance on God may be perceived as passive, their struggle to live and determine their futures are clear indicators of their choice to move with God "from victim to change agent."

After the initial pain and shock of the cancer diagnosis wears off, Black breast cancer survivors invariably focus on living. They undergo treatments, change their lifestyles, and make adjustments to remain cancer free. Although cancer recurrence is something breast cancer survivors think about, most believe that following their initial diagnoses and treatment, breast cancer is behind them. Yet, sometimes breast cancer returns or it spreads to other organs. At these times, cancer survivors face the inevitable truth that they will die from breast cancer. When Black breast cancer survivors face their own mortality and eminent death from breast cancer, they do so with resolve to live fully until the end. They trust God to take care of them even when no further conventional cancer treatments are available.

African American breast cancer survivors' resolve to live fully despite a terminal prognosis is not because they are unaware of what will happen. These cancer survivors are not in denial about the "facts" of their health, despite what some health-care providers might think. Neither are they in denial about the "facts" of death or their own mortality. Death, whether or not from breast cancer, is a part of life. Instead, when African American breast cancer survivors experience metastasis or are diagnosed as terminal, most make a conscious decision to resist. They chose to struggle against what breast cancer seeks to take from them—hope, joy, wholeness, and life.

Rather than acquiesce to breast cancer, Black breast cancer survivors challenge the injustice and indignities of breast cancer. They resist what breast cancer threatens to take from them, along with others' distorted ideas about their faith. Why they resist and how they resist reflect their theological perspectives about God and themselves. African American cancer survivors believe God stands for life and their well-being. Because God stands for life, anything that harms or takes life is not of God. Black breast cancer survivors therefore struggle against breast cancer because it is not the best they believe God intends for them. They resist death in particular by trusting God even more to take care of them.

African American cancer survivors' abilities to resist challenges that breast cancer presents, particularly questions about their faith with late-stage disease, are directly connected to African American women's history of social marginalization. Marginalized groups, including African American breast cancer survivors, often resist oppression through ideological and embodied struggles against power, hierarchy, and control. Demonstrated through what Scott calls everyday forms of resistance, marginalized groups who are otherwise socially and politically powerless regain power over their lives by challenging dominant paradigms about how poor and disenfranchised groups act in response to what harms them.[11] Rather than passively acquiesce, everyday forms of resistance subvert the naturalness of oppression, including stereotypes about how African American women react to breast cancer, by replacing them with non-elites counter-narratives.

These non-elite counter-narratives or what Black women believe about God in response to cancer oppose the ideological dominance of elite groups and their values, including those of medical professionals. While the medical community at large might view some African American breast cancer survivors' faith in God as ill-conceived with late-stage disease, this only makes Black cancer survivors rely on God more. Although African American breast cancer survivors have counter-narratives about God and poor cancer prognoses, they do not commonly express them to people in positions of authority, like health-care providers. Instead African American cancer survivors communicate offstage with family and friends what they truly believe through their offhand comments and conversations and through forms of expressive culture, like diaries or testimonies.[12] What African American breast cancer survivors believe about God and poor cancer prognoses that they do not share with their health-care providers are hidden transcripts. Hidden transcripts are counter-narratives that African American breast cancer survivors share outside of detection by elites.[13]

What African American breast cancer survivors believe about God, but do not share with their providers out of fear of being misinterpreted, happens in tandem with their public transcripts. Public transcripts are the open interactions elites and non-elites have with each other.[14] Public transcripts are the encounters African American breast cancer survivors have with their health-care providers who provide them with the facts of diagnose and treatment. These public transcripts usually maintain social hierarchies and unequal power dynamics common in stratified social contexts, including health-care settings.[15] Because African American cancer survivors do not openly resist health-care providers' misperceptions or stereotypes about them, often these ideas persist. Consequently, the hidden transcripts African American breast cancer survivors generate about God, poor cancer prognoses, and death only surface with deeper inquiry. With deeper inquiry, what becomes clear is that Black breast cancer survivors do not view relying on God as giving up. Instead relying on God is an active form of resistance against breast cancer. It is what transforms their pain into them effecting change in their lives. This is something Karla Atkins is well aware of.

Karla Atkins is a young, professional, African American woman and a breast cancer survivor.[16] Karla is well acquainted with breast cancer. While in her twenties, Karla's mother died from terminal breast cancer. Having lost a mother to breast cancer, Karla works at doing what she can to prevent a recurrence. Even though she has been cancer free for more than a decade, Karla is not unaware that people die from breast cancer. She saw it with her mother and experienced its devastating affects with her aunt.

For several years following her treatment, Karla tried to make sense of why she was diagnosed with breast cancer at such a young age. Her answer came with her maternal aunt's diagnosis.

> After I got breast cancer, my aunt got it, my mom's younger sister. Actually [my aunt] was her middle sister. And it was really interesting because she had a really hard time [after being diagnosed]. She just couldn't believe it. And it was at that point I really realized why I got it. Because I kept saying, "Why? Why did I get cancer at such a young age?" And when she got it, I immediately knew why. I felt like it was to help her through because she was having a tough time [with being diagnosed].

Karla's experience with breast cancer would help her guide her aunt through her experience with the disease. She had helped her aunt through other challenging situations. Karla resolved she would do the same with breast cancer.

Karla helped her aunt with making decisions about her breast cancer treatment by encouraging her aunt to opt for a mastectomy versus a lumpectomy. Karla also took her aunt to get chemotherapy and to be fitted with her breast prosthesis. At every step along the breast cancer journey Karla was there to encourage her aunt, reassuring her that she would survive breast cancer. Even after her aunt's treatment was finished, Karla continued to remind her aunt about maintaining healthy lifestyle choices to support her well-being. Karla was encouraging her aunt to resist recurrence by making intentional choices to live. Two years after her aunt's diagnosis, Karla believed her aunt would remain cancer free. However, the cancer came back. Karla remembered when she first noticed that something was wrong,

> And maybe two years later she started having pains in her side and in her hips. And she kept putting off going to the doctor. I said, "Meredith, you know you really need to go to the doctor." She put it off for several months. And I said [finally], "If you don't go to the doctor soon, I'm going to take off, make the appointment, and take you to the doctor because this is not good." She was like, "Oh, I'll do it after the wedding" because her daughter was getting married. I noticed that at the wedding, she really had some difficulties getting down the aisle. And I knew, at that point, I said, "Um um. Something's wrong. You need to make the appointment now. No more excuses." She made the appointment and she found out she had liver cancer. It had to be either at the end of June or early July.

Karla soon discovered that her aunt's breast cancer had metastasized and spread to her liver.

Although her aunt had experienced a recurrence, Karla assumed that, as before, she would successfully assist her aunt through her second bout with cancer. Accompanying her to chemotherapy and radiation treatments as she had done before, it soon became clear to Karla that her aunt's health was declining.

> She had been taking her medicine and she had to do some chemo and radiation [after her diagnosis in midsummer]. I was like, "Well okay. They can get it out. You'll be okay." But I noticed that her health started to decline. I was like, "Something's not right!" So I asked her if it would be okay if I would call her doctor. And she said, "For what?" And I said, "Well, I just want to talk to him and kind of see what's going on." So she finally said, "Okay."

Wanting to understand what was happening to her aunt, Karla finally persuaded her aunt to give her permission to speak with her oncologist. What her aunt's oncologist said surprised her. What he told her also reflected what he presumed about Karla's aunt and her perceived inability to grasp what was happening to her.

> So I talked to him and he said, "Her daughter has come with her and I'm not sure that she understands that she's not doing well." I said, "What do you mean?" And he said, "Well, I've told her that her health is declining. It's really spread. And it doesn't look good. But it doesn't seem to be clicking with her." I said, "What do you mean?" And he was like, "She doesn't seem to understand." And I said, "Well, she doesn't have trouble understanding. So clearly that's not it. She just may be taking a more positive outlook." He said, "I want to make sure that she understands what the prognosis is." And I said, "Well explain to me in layman's terms." And that's when he said, "Well, I don't think that she's going to last through the holidays." And I was like, "What?" And this was probably September.

Although Karla interpreted her aunt's reaction to her prognosis as one of maintaining hopefulness and choosing not to suffer with her recurrence, the oncologist viewed her aunt's response as one of confusion about the facts of her declining health. While the mismatch between how her aunt and her aunt's oncologist viewed the situation was obvious, what was more devastating for Karla was the prognosis. Her aunt was dying.

> The doctor gave her till Christmas [to survive]. And I mean I was just shocked. I was like, "What!" I mean I was just so in shock. I had a really, really hard time with it. And he [physician] finally told me this [in September] because I had been relying on her to get information back and forth.

At the same time that Karla found out her aunt was dying from breast cancer, she was also confronted with the reality of how quickly, based on the medical facts, she would succumb. Having been with her aunt throughout both cancer diagnoses and treatment, Karla was not prepared for her aunt's impending death.

Even though she was not initially prepared for her aunt's death, Karla quickly realized that she would help her aunt live until she died, just has she had helped her live through previous diagnosis and treatment. Karla remembered her conversation with her aunt shortly after she learned what her prognosis was,

> After [my talk with her doctor] I had a conversation with her. She was like, "You know, I'm not accepting this. You know, I've prayed about it. Whatever the Lord's will is, let it be done. But I know he has the power to heal me." So she kind of took that approach. She really started to have some problems when she started the radiation and the chemo because the chemo took all of her hair out. She had a really hard time with the hair loss and then her kids. Her kids, I think had somewhat of a detrimental effect on her. Because they were close to their mom they just couldn't take it [seeing her dying]. Every time they saw her, they would just burst into tears.

When Karla talked to her aunt she finally heard her aunt's hidden transcript about her prognosis. Karla's aunt believed that God would take care of her. She was willing to trust God's will for her life. Karla's aunt was also resolute in her faith that God's power could heal her and therefore she chose to live. Even as her health further declined, Karla's aunt continued to believe that God would be with her. She was not giving up on life. She was depending even more on God to see her through. Her act of resistance would be to live as long as possible. And Karla's aunt did persist.

Even when she became bedridden, Karla's aunt continued to resist death. Karla says,

> It got to a point where I kind of moved in with her, particularly on the weekends. If I couldn't be there, I would go there every night and stay with her. Help her get turned in bed. Make sure she had her medications. And I mean, at the time I was working full-time. I was up like every two hours with her because at that point she had become paralyzed, from the waist down, and she was in a wheel chair. After her treatments, she was just oh God, I mean really sick. She couldn't hold down water. She was really sick. But, fortunately we were able to keep her comfortable. Her younger sister, my Aunt Betty, we basically took care of her. Her son helped a lot. I kept her comfortable made, sure she got to the doctors. And I would splurge with her. Like she'd say, "You know, I have a taste for this," and I would go and get it. You know anything I could do to keep her spirits up and keep her comfortable. She actually passed away in June of the following year. She lasted. Yeah she lasted quite a few months longer than he [physician] expected.

Karla and her aunt struggled against breast cancer. Rather than let the disease take her joy, Karla helped her aunt manage her physical pain. They sought ways to keep her spirits up. Even as her health declined and she was actively dying, Karla's aunt was resisting. A consequence of this resistance was that Karla's aunt lived longer than what her doctor had predicted she would. Even while dying, Karla's aunt seemed determined to live until the very end.

Each day Aunt Meredith lived longer than what her doctor predicted was an act of resistance. She refused to accept death even when her cancer prognosis was not good. She chose to rely on faith in God to see her through. Meredith's hidden transcript, revealed to Karla, expressed Meredith's true beliefs about her prognosis and her response to it. Even though her health was declining, Meredith was not giving up. Although Meredith's oncologist assumed she did not understand what was happening to her, Meredith clearly understood. Meredith chose not to openly challenge her oncologist's public transcript about her—namely, misperceptions about what her complete faith in God meant. Instead Meredith chose to privately challenge the facts of her prognosis by focusing on living.

Meredith underwent treatment and did everything possible to live, trusting in God's ultimate will for her life. Karla supported her aunt's living and dying and affirmed her trust in God. For Karla's aunt and other Black breast cancer survivors like her, resistance even while dying is about trusting in God, the one who stands for life.

Other African American breast cancer survivors resist being labeled as fatalists because they trust in God and also refuse to give into breast cancer. While they know that breast cancer may be what they ultimately die from, they choose to live without fear of death. Refusing to fear death is also an act of resistance for some African American breast cancer survivors. For these survivors resisting death, by relinquishing control to God, what others may call fatalism is the only way to live. This is what Carlice Harris believes.[17] Her resisting breast cancer by choosing to be unafraid of death is a process, one that took some time for her to come to.

When Carlice was initially diagnosed, she at first thought about death. She thought about pain, suffering, and dying. Well-being was not what she initially thought about. She thought about those she knew who had died from cancer and how they had suffered.

> And you see everybody that you have seen die with cancer. You see that. You see these folks that you have seen who had cancer. And oftentimes it's like they wasted away. [They] got real small. They couldn't eat. They were nauseated and couldn't keep nothing down. And that's what comes to you. The bad part comes to you when they say "cancer." Healing and well-being is not what you're thinking about. You're thinking about probably that worst side. You're thinking of the worst side right then. So you deny that. You say, "I can't see myself like that." And then you say, "Yeah. That's what it's going to be because he [physician] just told me that 'you have cancer.'" That's what it is going to be [illness, suffering, and death].

Carlice, like a lot of African American women who are diagnosed with breast cancer, thought about the worst. Carlice description of what she experienced parallels Lorde's ideas about suffering. Carlice, once diagnosed, suffered.

Yet what changed Carlice's perspective (i.e., moved her from suffering to being transformed by her pain) was seeing another breast cancer survivor. When she interacted with a representative from the American Cancer Society she realized that while some do die from breast cancer, not all Black women diagnosed with cancer die. Many Black women live. It was interacting with another Black cancer survivor that changed her perspective. It gave her something to aspire to. It is something she wishes all African American women diagnosed with breast cancer had.

> I think one of the keys [to changing a breast cancer survivor's outlook] is that something could come into your life or eyesight or something to move you from that. If you just had something [hopeful to aspire toward]. But, I'm sure that that does not happen to every woman. She doesn't get the bright side early enough. And somebody to just come in and tell her, "Hey. You don't have to dwell on the dark side. There is more than one side."

When Carlice started thinking about other women she knew who had survived breast cancer, it started her to really thinking about life, death, and pain. Her thinking refocused by the pain of having breast cancer, in combination with her faith, developed her resistive consciousness.

As Carlice thought deeply about the pain of breast cancer she realized that death even from breast cancer was not something to be feared. Not fearing death from breast cancer has been key to Carlice's well-being. Her lack of fear also serves to challenge ideas about African Americans and cancer fatalism.

> There's one thing that I have learned since I have had breast cancer: In order for me to enjoy living that I should no longer be afraid of dying. It has taught me not to be afraid of dying. I cannot really enjoy living [until I'm no longer afraid of death]. And I'm enjoying living. [But,] I couldn't enjoy living the way I enjoy living if I was worried about and afraid of dying. And so you learn not to be afraid of dying. And that takes some study [of your spirituality]. It takes some understanding on your part. And that takes some dedication on your part. And when you learn that you say, "Well. Hey, this is something that is coming [death]." I just want to be ready to deal with it because it's coming whether I have cancer or not. It [death] is coming. And it's going to take care of itself. So my job is to learn to think of it in the way I ought to think of it [as something to not worry about, but prepare for].

Instead of being afraid of death and suffering as a consequence, Carlice has made peace with death. Death is a part of life, something outside of her absolute control. Death is a reality that comes with having breast cancer. Carlice's accepting this fact is not resignation or fatalism. Her accepting the reality of death is the starting point for her living. She has undergone what Townes calls moving from "victim to change agent." Refusing to be afraid of breast cancer and death struggles against breast cancer and what it seeks to take from Carlice and other Black women—namely, their hope, faith, and life itself. When Carlice refuses to fear death she no longer fears breast cancer. That is the hidden transcript she operates with and the one that makes all the difference for her well-being.

When it comes to breast cancer and the odds of long-term survival, the odds are not stacked in Black women's favor. With higher mortality rates from breast cancer, a greater likelihood of being diagnosed at younger ages, and subject to more lethal forms of the disease, African American women have a right to be pessimistic about surviving breast cancer, even to the point of being fatalistic. However, when Black women's acceptance of death and trust in God's will are presumed to mean that they have given up on life or are out of touch with reality, this is where the problem lies. For what African American women with breast cancer actual believe often belies what others, including some health-care providers, think about Black women's theology and their responses to terminal breast cancer diagnoses and death. What Black women truly believe usually only surfaces in their hidden transcripts and not their public encounters with their health-care providers.

In the face of odds that are stacked against them, African American breast cancer survivors persist to live. They persist because they think about dying from breast cancer the same way they think about living with breast cancer. They believe God is with them. Because God is with them, death is not something to fear. Breast cancer is not something to suffer from. Both are to be resisted because of what they steal—hope, wholeness, their well-being and life itself.

The fact of breast cancer for these African American cancer survivors is that it is a disease that takes away and diminishes life. It is a disease that can bring both pain and suffering. Pain is something they can work with. Suffering is not. In response to both pain and suffering they construct God as one who stands for life and its flourishing. Jesus's resurrection provided the victory over suffering. Therefore, when Black women rely on God throughout diagnosis and treatment, and come to depend even more on God with recurrence and death, they are being true to their theology and faith. Their theology tells them that suffering is sin because it seeks remedy from pain without God. Their theology also tells them that pain, when examined, can be used for transformation. With God, they can struggle with pain by moving from being a victim of breast cancer to a change agent in response to breast cancer. As a change agent, Black women with breast cancer make plans about their future and how they will live it—not in accordance to, but in response to the disease and its facts.

It is this theology, one that does not accept breast cancer as God's will, that supports Black women's faith. Their faith in God is what compels them to believe they have come too far with God to turn back now, even if it means facing death. So when African American breast cancer survivors live despite the odds against them and keep living to their fullest until they die, their very survival is an act of resistance—resistance against the disease, the facts of the disease, other's misperceptions of them, fatalism, and everything else breast cancer tries to take from them.

NOTES

1. Gerend, M., and Pai, M. (2008). "Social Determinants of Black-White Disparities in Breast Cancer Mortality: A Review." *Cancer Epidemiology, Biomarkers & Prevention, 17* (11): 2913–2923.
2. Newman, L., and Kaljee, L. (2017). "Health Disparities and Triple-Negative Breast Cancer in African American Women: A Review." *JAMA Surgery*, 485–493.
3. Yedjou, C., et al. (2017). Assessing the Racial and Ethnic Disparities in Breast Cancer Mortality in the United States." *International Journal of Environmental Research and Public Health, 14* (486): 1–14.
4. Gerend and Pai. "Social Determinants of Black-White Disparities in Breast Cancer Mortality"; Lannin, D., Mathews, H., Mitchell, J., Swanson, M., Swanson, F., and Edwards, M. (1998). "Influence of Socioeconomic Status and Cultural Factors on Racial Differences in Late-Stage Presentation of Breast Cancer." *JAMA, 279*, 1801–1807; and Skinner, C., Arfken, C., and Sykes, R. (1998). "Knowledge, Perceptions, and Mammography Stage of Adoption among Older Urban Women." *American Journal of Preventive Medicine, 14*, 54–63.
5. Powe, B., Daniels, E., and Finnie, R. (2005). "Comparing Perceptions of Cancer Fatalism among African American Patients and Their Providers." *Journal of the Academy of Nursing Practice*, 318–324.
6. Drew, E., and Schoenberg, N. (2011). "Deconstructing Fatalism: Ethnographhc Perspectives on Women's Decision Making about Cancer Prevention and Treatment." *Medical Anthropology Quarterly, 25* (2): 164–182.
7. Morgan, P., Tyler, I., and Fogel, J. (2008). "Fatalism Revisited." *Seminars in Oncology Nursing*, 237–245; and Tate, J. (2011). "The Role of Spiritualty in the Breast Cancer Experiences of African American Women." *Journal of Holistic Nursing, 29* (4): 249–255.
8. Lorde, A. (1984). "Eye to Eye: Black Women, Hatred, and Anger." In *Sister Outsider*, 171–172. Trumansburg, NY: Crossing Press.
9. Townes, E. (Ed.). (1993). "Living in the New Jerusalem: The Rhetoric and Movement of Liberation in the House of Evil." In *A Troubling in My Soul: Womanist Perspectives on Evil & Suffering*, 78–91. Maryknoll, NY: Orbis Books.
10. Ibid., 84.
11. Scott, J. (1985). *Weapons of the Weak: Everyday Forms of Peasant Resistance.* New Haven, CT: Yale University Press.
12. Ibid.
13. Ibid.
14. Ibid.
15. Ibid.
16. Karla Atkins is a pseudonym and personal details of her life have been fictionalized.
17. Carlice Harris is a pseudonym and personal details of her life have been fictionalized.

II

Black Women Respond to God and Breast Cancer

Chapter Five

Black Women Transformed into Cancer Survivors

When Black women have experienced a life-changing experience like breast cancer, how they view life is never the same as it was before. In many ways breast cancer is like a religious conversion experience for some African American women. Identifying with the crucified and resurrected Jesus Christ, life before diagnosis and the suffering Black women endure through treatment gives way to something new, during and after cancer treatment. As Townes says, God's breaking into humanity through the resurrection transforms these Black women's "suffering into wholeness" moving them from "victim to change agent."[1] This was something I heard repeatedly from African American breast cancer survivors. For cancer survivors, who they are and what they do after the cancer diagnosis changes. They are no longer victims of breast cancer. They are change agents because of breast cancer. And while some African American breast cancer survivors attempt to resume their pre-cancer-diagnosis lives, others are not content with just surviving breast cancer. For the latter, their experiences with breast cancer spur them to want to be and do more.

For survivors who desire more following their cancer diagnosis, resuming life as they were before the diagnosis is out of the question. They have seen too much and experienced far too much. The prospect of getting back to an old "normal" seems too small a reward for having faced, struggled with, and survived breast cancer. These survivors endow the breast cancer survivorship experience with greater meaning and more socially redemptive purposes than just surviving.

Breast cancer necessitates for many African American breast cancer survivors, the experience's use for a greater good. Survival creates opportunities for new perspectives on living, even at times requiring new and radically different ways of being well. Having faced death, many African American cancer survivors become particularly determined to celebrate the fact they are alive. These survivors refuse just to survive cancer. They instead want to thrive in spite of breast cancer. Thriving beyond breast cancer becomes a focal point for well-being. This thriving also influences how Black cancer survivors use their agency to help themselves and others.

As I became increasingly aware of the diverse ways African American breast cancer survivors use their experiences to act and live in new ways, I also identified a framework for identifying and describing African American cancer survivors' agency during survivorship. Porter's text, *Leading Ladies: Transformative Biblical Images for Women's Leadership*, provided this framework.[2] Particularly, it identifies Black women's agency as culturally influenced and manifested forms of leadership. African American breast cancer survivors' agency mapped onto these female biblical models reflects "leadership" in the truest sense of the word. At the heart of the word leadership is the root word "to go."[3]

Not just a command "to go," the term "leadership" implies that one has the capacity to guide others along a path (or through an experience) as a consequence of having traveled there before. African American cancer survivors in this study had often been placed in situations to motivate and care for others (especially in the context of cancer) because they had experienced cancer themselves. Not only have these survivors faced cancer, they have thrived even beyond it. Their living and thriving are the basis for their authority to act as leaders. These African American breast cancer survivors reflect what the anthropologist Susan Shinagawa terms as "thrivers."[4]

African American breast cancer survivors are heirs to a rich, historical tradition of Black women, one in which the intersections of race, class, and gender have required Black women to survive against seemingly insurmountable odds. Additionally, because of their cancer diagnoses, these African American cancer survivors have also faced their own mortality. These women live with the ever-present reminder that death is a part of life. They face the possibility of death every time they go for another mammogram, test, or doctor's appointment. Although they are often afraid, "thrivers" choose to move beyond fear and to use whatever time remains to make a tangible difference for themselves and others.

African American cancer survivors' decisions to act as leaders are influenced by their ever-evolving self-definitions of who they are as breast cancer survivors. Their understanding of self is in keeping with self-defined Black women's standpoint and Black feminist/womanist ways of seeing the world. Indicative of Black female leadership, as African American breast cancer survivors search for their own healing, they use what they learn to support the well-being of others in their community.[5] African American breast cancer survivors' self-awareness not only defines who they are, but also influences their relationships with others, including God. In this context, consequently, "leadership" serves as shorthand for identifying roles African American breast cancer survivors use throughout their survivorship to make a difference.

Using Porter's ideas about leadership offers a new epistemological way of approaching Black breast cancer survivors' agency. Porter's leadership model identifies female biblical archetypes as ways to identify African American survivors' diverse styles of action in response to breast cancer. Porter's "leading ladies" reflect the thriving spirit evidenced in African American breast cancer survivor's narratives. These roles also provide ways to understand the behavioral motivations behind how Black survivors respond to breast cancer. Leadership and these female archetypical roles function as ways to describe African American breast cancer survivors' activities and actions. Considering Black breast cancer survivors' agency against female biblical actors as womanist models for leadership requires locating women's leadership in the broader context of the history of political thought and feminist /womanist debates about leadership and women as leaders.

WOMEN AS LEADERS: THOUGHTS, DEBATES, AND FEMINIST/WOMANIST CRITIQUES

Ideas about women as leaders have coincided with larger philosophical questions, throughout the seventeenth to twentieth centuries, about representation and the obligations of human beings to each other in society. As such, this has made tracing the history of feminist theories of leadership a somewhat complicated one.[6] The lack of distinct feminist theories of leadership, up until relatively recently in the twentieth to twenty-first centuries, stems from the nature of feminism itself. Leadership has primarily focused on public life, which has been dominated by men. Women and their roles, in contrast, have been relegated to the domestic sphere, including family and social relations. Because feminism rose in opposition to male-dominated and masculine forms of power, feminists, by nature, have been ambivalent toward leadership and power.[7]

While, as Vetter points out, it takes leadership to advance the causes that achieve equity for women, leadership as it has been traditionally conceived as masculine and authoritarian has not well served the needs of women.[8] As a result, feminist thinkers, both in theory and practice, have had to wrestle with, challenge, and question ideas of power, citizenship, autonomy, and representation inherent to leadership, which have come from the broader history of political thought—a history often dominated by men. As a consequence, identifying women's leadership roles and feminist/womanist theorizing about leadership have been oppositional in nature and critical in response to how women have been conceived by social thinkers as change agents. A brief history of key political ideas that shape feminist/womanist ideas about leadership and that influence how Black women assert their agency as breast cancer survivors is needed.

One of the earliest thinkers regarding people as social agents was John Locke. In his work, *Second Treatise on Civil Government*, Locke describes a hypothetical state of nature as one in which males and females, as self-interested beings, defend themselves against each other.[9] It is on the basis of this principle of self-preservation that humans, as rational beings, make calculated decisions to consent to political rule and other associations, including institutions like marriage.

The state of nature Locke hypothesizes conceivably provides the basis for freedom and equality, yet in actuality, people are unable to live without overarching structure. It response, Locke theorized that humans consent to form governments that allow for representation and protection from threats in exchange for giving up some of their self-interested rights. Governments and their representatives (i.e., leaders) are expected to uphold the basic rights of their constituents in order to remain in power. If governments (and leaders) fail to uphold their responsibilities to their constituents, then governments (and leaders) can be overthrown and new ones established. This is the basis of the social contract.[10]

Locke's ideas about the relative egalitarianism of society have proven limiting for women's participation in the public sphere and for feminist theories of leadership, which have emerged to challenge it. Locke's claims about the conjugal basis of marriage are based on gender inequality. Locke believed that because women were less capable of defending themselves while pregnant, they had to depend on men for protection.[11] Therefore Locke's natural egalitarianism between men and women falls apart because in actuality, rather than have equal footing in making decisions, husbands (and by extension men) are "abler and stronger" than their wives (and by extension women) and therefore are the last word in settling disputes.[12] Locke's ideas about unequal power dynamics among domestic partners is one that feminist theorists and activists challenged over the centuries.

Jean-Jacques Rousseau questioned Locke's ideas about freedom and equality in the state of nature. Nevertheless, he was also interested in the elements of a just and equitable society. In particular Rousseau believed that representatives (i.e., leaders) should be held directly accountable to their constituents upon penalty of death.[13] While Rousseau's ideas about the functioning of society held out hope for women's having greater opportunities for leadership, Rousseau's work backtracks from this possibility, instead carving out a separate and seemingly equal role for women.[14] As Rousseau imagined, women should receive an education that was fundamentally different from that of men.[15] Women's education would teach them to be the moral guarantors of society, charged with rearing morally upright children and using their powers of sexual manipulation to maintain their households and keep ethically wayward spouses in check.[16] As with Locke, Rousseau's ideas about women's proscribed roles as leaders, those who exert influence over others, would also be critiqued by later generations of feminist scholars.

Thinkers in both the nineteenth and twentieth centuries provided ways of thinking that have significantly informed feminist theorizing about leadership. With the rise in the nineteenth century of revolutions in Europe, and abolitionism and the women's suffrage movements in the United States, possibilities for the greater rights for women were seemingly on the horizon. Karl Marx's ideas, affected by these social movements, offered new ways of thinking about oppression, particularly in relation to property rights.[17] His ideas in *The Communist Manifesto* about the inequitable relationship between the dominant group or bourgeoisie, who owned the means of production, and the systematic oppression of the proletariat, the workers who sold their labor, laid bare that the only means of addressing these inequities was through social revolution. Advocating for a communal way of life, free from management, Marx outlined a type of state that would conceivably allow for women to emerge as political leaders, although he never explicitly called for this.[18]

In the twentieth century, the French philosopher Michel Foucault is largely responsible for shaping political theory about power and authority, which are central to leadership. His ideas regarding how those with power use knowledge, religion, and social institutions to dominate others and how those who are "othered" respond to their domination were core ideas. Emphasizing the perspectives of those who are marginalized and silenced (e.g., criminals, homosexuals), Foucault emphasized the ways in which power operates in society as what he terms "mechanisms of power."[19] Naming groups of people is a discursive mechanism of power. Those who create the dominant discourse define themselves in relation to how they differ from those they construct as "other" (e.g., controlling images of Black women). Those who are constructed as "other" by the dominant discourse internalize these views and use them for their own purposes (e.g., Strong Black Woman schema). Discourse, as Foucault described, was related to another mechanism of power called the "panopticon," "the gaze," or the power of surveillance. Dominant groups' abilities to name and scrutinize others, Foucault argued, was so totalizing that once instituted, the marginalized regulated their own behavior in accordance to their surveillance.[20] Although Foucault's work does not focus on women, his thoughts on the discursive use of gender as an arbitrary mechanism have been useful to feminists in reclaiming women's marginalized discourse and using it to frame debates that affect women's lives.

The work of these thinkers in the twentieth and twenty-first centuries has given shape to feminist theories of leadership of three distinct kinds. One is what is called the "ethic of care." Building on Rousseau's ideas about the complementary roles or men and women, yet seeking not to reinforce inequalities between the sexes, an ethics of care as a feminist theory of women's leadership has expanded feminine virtues like compassion and caring, which have long been seen as part of women's work in the domestic sphere, and applied these to women's leadership in political life and the public sphere.[21] Joan Tronto, a major feminist theorist, redefines care as both a disposition and action to reach out to other people in society at large.[22] Female leaders who evidence an ethics of care in their styles of leadership evidence an attentiveness to the needs of others: a sense of responsibility, obligations, and duties necessitated by the contexts in which they are working; competence in executing desired ends and results; and responsiveness to those receiving care. Female leaders who operate out of an ethic of care also manifest integrity of care, which brings these elements together by reconciling conflicts between them.[23]

Not to reinforce negative feminine stereotypes, but to challenge ideas about men's leadership styles, other feminist theorists of leadership have proposed the "Great Woman" theory of leadership.[24] The focus of this work is on female leaders who are "collaborative, cooperative, supportive, understanding, gentle, emotional and vulnerable."[25] These qualities are offered as counterpoint to the "Great Man" theories of leadership, which value traits associated with men in power, like dominance, confidence, reason, charisma, determination, and other masculine characteristics.[26] As a part of this theory of leadership, women are also noted for having greater emotional intelligence, as well as the ability to perceive, respond to, and manage emotions more effectively in work settings.[27] While women as leaders may reflect these characteristics, women who do not conform to these traits may suffer backlash or be excluded from positions that do not easily lend themselves to these traits.[28]

Feminist theorists influenced by Foucault's ideas about power, discourse, and surveillance have critically examined how women's oppression is tied to formal and informal institutions, cultural discourses, and social practices. Foucault-informed feminist theories of leadership consider how power in leadership discourse holds women back, particularly if the individuals who are the subjects of analyses are overwhelmingly male. Critical feminist theories of leadership look for mechanisms of power at the micro-level to understand how they are detrimental to women at the macro-level.[29] Such scholarship offers the potential for creating alternative discourse that empowers women and their leadership. Marion Young's feminist alternatives to leadership emphasize leadership that is participatory, egalitarian, and democratic. Young takes as a given that political discourse does not operate on a level playing field for all involved, thus recognizing that inequalities in exercising leadership persist for women and people of color.[30] She therefore insists on an all-inclusive approach to political discourse that moves beyond privileging formal rational argument as the sole means of political debate to include personal narratives, testimonies, and storytelling as equally valid forms of political discourse.[31]

In addition to reframing the tools of political discourse, Young also outlines a feminist theory of representation as a model of leadership.[32] In this approach leaders are representatives who reflect the interests, opinions and perspectives of their constituents. The interests of the people being represented may not be the self-interests of the representative, whose perspectives are shaped by experiences, personal and social histories, over time. The interests that the representative puts forth may also not be synonymous with the opinions, values, or priorities that the individual leader holds. Therefore, a leader sublimates her interests for the good of the greater whole.[33] What these contemporary feminist theories of leadership have done is lift up the gendered ways leaders operate and how women as leaders execute their power out of collective interest, rather than self-interest, in service to others. This work has been useful to both feminist scholarship and activism. However, this work also has its critics.

Calling out the ways mainstream feminist discourse has further marginalized Black women and other women of color, twentieth-century Black feminists like bell hooks have used Marx's ideas to critique white bourgeois politics in mainstream feminism, which advocates for greater equity for privileged white women to the exclusion of women of color and for all people.[34] Patricia Hill Collins, in line with Foucault's ideas about institutional power and how discourse marginalizes people, has examined how race, class, and gender have been used to oppress African American women (i.e., controlling images). Collins's work in particular advocates for a distinct Black women's standpoint as a starting point for examining Black women's roles in the public sphere, including as leaders.[35] Black women's operation as leaders emerged out of the historical necessity of Black women to not only contend with sexism from Black men, but also race, sex, and class oppression from whites. In response to these oppressions, Black women created safe havens within Black communities for personal and collective survival, which developed into a "cultural of political resistance" that required Black women to expand their roles as homemakers and workers to become "caretakers of the race."[36] The cultivation and operationalization of Black female leadership, therefore, took place within the leaders' roles in family and community (i.e., churches, schools, political organizations).[37]

Further challenging feminist theories about women as a monolithic cultural group, critical race theorist Kimberle Crenshaw coined the term "intersectionality" as a metaphor to explain how women of color are affected by multiple systems of oppression, marked by race, gender, and class differentials, without being recognized for their unique experiences at the convergence of these systems.[38] By considering the convergence of identities, as Smooth points out, "intersectionality posits that race, class, gender, sexuality, ability and various aspects of identity are constitutive. Each informs the other, and taken together they produce a way of experiencing the world as sometimes oppressed and marginalized and sometimes privileged and advantaged depending on the context."[39] This insight is beneficial to theories about Black women's leadership because it recognizes that power is dynamic and shifting, rather than static, absolute, and fixed. Black women's exercise of leadership shifts in accordance to the social dynamics they experience. Their experiences as leaders are not shaped only by their race or their gender, but by the convergence of their identities.

Because organizations (and society at large) are not race, gender, or class neutral, Black women who are different from the norm in organizations and institutions (e.g., by virtue of being female in the male dominated Black church or civil rights organizations, etc.) have often faced marginalization or invisibility, which seemingly run counter to their roles as leaders.[40] Given that this is true, feminist/womanist scholars have reconsidered how Black women's leadership is exercised. Historian Belinda Robnett's examination of leadership in the civil rights movement demonstrated how using common definitions of leadership, including those that mark leadership as being the public face of organizations and speaking in front of crowds, overlooks the less public contributions of Black women as leaders. She argues that continuing to use models of leadership that have centered on how men perform leadership will result in leaders who were women of color going unnoticed.[41] What critiques of leadership historiography have led to is a closer examination of women of color's experiences to determine what shapes women of color's leadership and the leadership roles these women play.

Patricia Hill-Collins also documents one of the sites where Black women gain epistemological perspective as leaders. She calls spaces where Black women, as part of marginalized groups, have traditionally been restricted from and yet have gained access to, as spaces where Black women operate as the "outsider within." Outsiders within are present in these spaces (e.g., Black domestics in white households, Black women academics in traditionally white, male-dominated university departments), yet they are not fully included or recognized as insiders. African American women who occupy this liminal space cultivate a critical view of dominant culture and are able to "see the contradictions between the dominant group's actions and ideologies."[42] Black women who are caught between groups of unequal power by virtue of their access to dominant groups, yet simultaneously retained marginalized identities, survive in these spaces by learning how to negotiate multiple systems of power. This is what informs their leadership and how they exercise it.

Robnett similarly documents how African American women's positions as women in the South during the civil rights movement was another strategic site for Black women's leadership and the roles they played. She calls African American women active in the movement "bridge leaders."[43] Given the South's gender politics of the 1950s and 1960s, women were seen as less threatening to the white dominant social class. As a consequence, African American women were able to take risks that African American men were not. As a result of Black women's operating under the radar of white repression, they were more often able to use their grassroots connections and social networks in communities and link them to formal civil rights organizations and their efforts. What also made these Black women successful as bridge leaders was their ability to link "strategies (aimed at individual change, identity, and consciousness) and political strategies (aimed at organizational tactics designed to challenge existing relationships with the state and other social institutions)."[44] Although their contributions have often been overlooked in historiography of the civil rights movement, these Black women's abilities to move between spaces and strategically use their relationships were key to the success of the movement in organizing local, grassroots politics.

Within the Black church, African American women's leadership has also often been overlooked. Because until the twentieth century most Black churches, because of sexism, denied women access to the pulpit, African American women nevertheless found ways to connect their religious beliefs to their activism and leadership. One of the earliest Black female preachers and evangelists, abolitionist Sojourner Truth, in her famous speech *Ain't I a Woman*, challenged the theology of opponents who claimed that women didn't deserve as many rights as men because Christ was a man. Truth in response countered saying, "Where did your Christ come from? From God and a Woman! Man had nothing to do with Him!"[45] Other historians like Cheryl Gilkes have excavated the contributions of Black women in the development and sustenance of the Black church, noting that outspoken women like Nannie Helen Burroughs, who was instrumental in organizing women's days within Black congregations and elevating the role of Black women as missionaries in the National Baptist Convention, as an exemplar of Black women's church-based leadership.[46] Womanist theologians like Renita Weems have used biblical texts to examine Black women's unequal social relations to white women and white feminist theology, using the story of Hagar and Sarah as an example.[47] Still other womanist theologians like Jacquelyn Grant and Delores Williams have sought to empower Black women through their analyses of biblical texts that tell the stories of powerful women in the bible as leaders and how their intersectional identities shaped their theology and responses of faith.[48]

As a critique of earlier centuries of political thought, which limited women's identities as both women and leaders, feminist/womanist scholars have challenged notions of democracy, egalitarianism, power, and equality embedded in ideas about leadership. Further offering correctives to masculine models of leadership, which emphasize charisma, determination, confidence, and other masculine traits, feminist/womanist theorists have theorized women's leadership based on enculturated female qualities like cooperation, collaboration, emotional intelligence, and an ethic of caring. These theories of women's leadership have served to elevate women's cultural features of leadership by putting them on equal footing with men's leadership. This has been helpful to both scholarship and activism. Yet, as liberating as this work has been, its benefits have not been equally shared by all women.

The idea that leadership is something all women equally exercise or benefit from is something Black feminist/womanist and critical race scholars in particular have pushed back against. Arguing that Black women and other women of color do not experience the world in the same way as white women, these scholars have called for a critical examination of the intersectionality of Black women's lives. The realities of race, gender, class, and other identities do not shape the experiences of Black women in an additive, but convergent, way. Because Black women cannot be reduced to either being Black or being female, who they are and how they are perceived in the world shapes their leadership, as it does other aspects of their lives. Consequently, this calls for (re)thinking about Black leadership in some new ways.

These new ways of (re)thinking Black women's leadership have called for abandoning masculine models of leadership when considering African American women's contributions to social movements. Instead of looking for top-down and publicly demonstrative styles of leadership, these scholars of Black women's leadership have looked at how Black women negotiate power as leaders by expanding their roles as homemakers and laborers to become "caretakers of the race" and by moving between spaces and serving as bridges between communities and organizations, linking individual identity and consciousness with challenging relationships with social institutions and existing power structures. Black women do this within their social networks, their communities, as well as within the Black church.

Exercising leadership within the Black church, African American women have repeatedly joined their faith to their activism. Whether as crusaders for social justice who used a womanist theology to counter patriarchal ideas of the primacy of men's rights over women's or as reformers within the church advocating for the public recognition of Black women as leaders, African American women have used church-based leadership as a way of asserting their ideas about egalitarianism, democracy, equality, and power and to challenge sexism within the Black church. Black women, as part of the Black church tradition, have also turned to biblical scriptures to shape the cultural hermeneutics of their social and political situations as Black women in relation to the world around them, finding there examples of biblical women who faced marginalization and oppression. In these same examples of biblical women, Black women scholars and non-scholars alike have also found models of leadership that resonate with their experiences and inform their activism.

LEADING LADIES: TRANSFORMATIVE WOMEN'S LEADERSHIP ROLES

Porter's transformative leadership roles indicative of Black feminist/womanist theoretical traditions present in the Black Church tradition recognize African American women as leaders, whether or not they have been termed as such. Predominant views of leadership, as have been described, have tended to favor masculine strategies of social engagement, such as "taking charge" or "giving orders." Usual Western leadership paradigms present "leaders always [as] seeming to be doing something *to* others, rarely doing things *with* others."[49] These culturally masculine ways of viewing leadership have resulted in other types of cultural leaders and cultural leadership styles being overlooked. As well, dominant scholarly approaches have reinforced ignoring women's leadership due to a focus on "key" historical figures and personalities (usually male), consequently rendering invisible most African American women's agency.

Rectifying these omissions in predominant leadership paradigms requires reconsidering leadership in light of African American breast cancer survivors' experiences. Doing this requires examining the lived realities of Black women and the ways they envision the world around them. Porter's transformative leadership model[50] achieves these ends. Based on Black feminist/womanist, self-defined women's standpoint and perspectives, these leadership roles also reflect a womanist "spirituality of survival."[51] They also are in line with the work of womanist theologians like Renita Weems and Delores Williams who have used the experiences of female biblical actors as reference points for explaining the experiences of contemporary Black women.

What makes these transformative leadership roles useful is that they provide tangible expressions of African American women's agency. They also evidence resources African American breast cancer survivors use to nurture their well-being and to cope with circumstances cancer presents (e.g., surgeries, treatment, life disruptions). By reimaging African American breast cancer survivors' agency as identifiable forms of leadership, even demoralizing circumstances survivors face can be reconsidered in light of the productive role they play in shaping survivors' well-being and others' well-being.

These leadership roles also function as a cultural resource for Black women touched by cancer, particularly those who self-identify as Christian, by providing biblical models for their agency. Porter's leadership roles (re)confirm God's presence in African American breast cancer survivors' day-to-day struggles for survival. These transformative leadership roles, and archetypes on which they are based, evidence for many African American breast cancer survivors God's dual roles as "liberator" and "judge," described in an earlier chapter. They also signify Jesus's relevance as a divine "cosufferer," who inspires them to stand for justice and healing.[52]

Through these roles, God intervenes in Black cancer survivor's lives. Survivors' ongoing communication with God prompts them to respond. African American survivors, in turn, respond in part by exercising leadership for others and themselves, similar to what Tronto calls an ethic of care.[53] Implicit in each of the leadership roles Porter sets forth is love as the ethical impetus for struggle and action.[54] The kind of active love evidenced in both Porter's work and Black feminist and womanist theoretical traditions, is supported by Christian ideals regarding charity and support. Love, demonstrated through charity and support for others, is often borne out of contentious circumstances.[55] "Love," or what the womanist ethicist Stacey Floyd-Thomas calls traditional communalism, is defined as "Black women's ability to create, re-member, nurture, protect, sustain and liberate."[56] For African American breast cancer survivors, love evidenced as traditional communalism sometimes requires personal discomfort and self-sacrifice in order to bring about sustained and beneficial change for self and others.

The goal of sustainable and beneficial change for others and self, as a manifestation of African American cancer survivors' well-being, provides the final parallel between Porter's role models and Black feminist/womanist thought. Porter never uses the words "wholeness" or "well-being" in her discussion. Nor does she explicitly mention the physical and materially felt aspects of transformative leadership or the roles she offers. Nevertheless, these sentiments are clearly evident in these roles.

Defining "transformative leadership," Porter envisions it as "the movement of people toward collective and mutual goals of spiritual growth, higher purpose, and empowerment."[57] Based in part on transformative leadership theories, notably as evidenced by Burns[58] and Bennis and Nanus,[59] Porter's implicit articulation of wholeness, manifested in transformative leadership, is based on the biblical principle Porter identifies as "transformation."

This notion of "transformation" as a precursor to leadership is most clearly evidenced for Porter (2000) in the scripture Romans 12: 1–2 (NLT). This scripture written by the apostle Paul states,

> And so I plead with you to give your bodies to God. Let them be a living and holy sacrifice—the kind he will accept. When you think of what he has done

for you, is this too much to ask? Don't copy the behavior and customs of this world, but let God transform you into a new person by changing the way you think. Then you will know what God wants you to do.

Transformative leadership, based on one's relationship with God and/or reliance upon a "spirituality of survival," first brings about struggle for wholeness within the African American breast cancer survivor herself; struggle borne out of her desire to survive cancer. In seeking to resolve her internal struggles with breast cancer, survivors seek God for reassurance and to make meaning from cancer. They entrust their bodies and cancer circumstances to God. These African American survivors believe that since God has been with them in other situations, God will also support them through breast cancer.

This relational experience consequently affects the way Black cancer survivors think. A change in the way they think, refashioned by a divinely determined love for self and others, provides a new way of perceiving (read as "standpoint") the world, situations, and others' behavior. Even things ostensibly antithetical and harmful to one's best interests (e.g., racism, sexism, breast cancer, etc.) are perceived differently than they were prior to breast cancer. Instead of seeing these oppressive and threatening situations as roadblocks, survivors come to view them as struggles God intends to teach them how to overcome.

A change in the way African American survivors perceive why cancer happens also necessitates a change in their own behaviors and ways of dealing with others. Through the experience of breast cancer and their social support seeking, African American cancer survivors are transformed. They become qualitatively different from how they knew themselves prior to diagnosis. Their transformation while experiencing cancer equips these African American survivors with power and abilities they previously were either unaware of or felt they did not possess.

African American breast cancer survivors become empowered through their cancer experiences. Because breast cancer changes their perspectives on dying, their thinking about living changes also. These Black cancer survivors become more clear and definite about their actions. Their actions are generally purposeful and confident. Their expressed leadership—namely, by helping others—takes on new and added meaning for these African American survivors. African American breast cancer survivors' intentional use of agency to make situations better for others and themselves is what Floyd-Thomas refers to as a womanist "moral anthropology."[60] "Moral anthropology" as she defines it is "the epistemological privilege of Black women knowing themselves and [that] their world stands under the moral imperative of making themselves and their world morally better."[61] Black breast cancer survivors believe that having survived breast cancer empowers them to make their world better.

LIVING OUT LOUD: CANCER SURVIVORS' LEADERSHIP

Breast cancer is a very real threat to African American cancer survivors' physical, spiritual, and psychosocial well-being. Breast cancer threatens life itself. Cancer changes how many African American breast cancer survivors think about and perceive the world around them. The value and meaning of things, such as time and opportunity, are altered forever. The experience also affects how African American breast cancer survivors perceive themselves and what they do. All of these issues Taylor very convincingly describes in her process-based model of breast cancer transformation.[62] The point where Porter's transformative leadership roles proves instructive is after Taylor's transformation phases have occurred in the lives of African American women affected by breast cancer. The weaver as one of Porter's leadership roles will be considered. Extending Porter's epistemological framework, the "seeking healer" role, which supports well-being, is offered as another breast cancer leadership role evident for some Black breast cancer survivors.

WEAVERS—LESSONS OF A LEADER

A weaver is a person who turns disparate materials into beautiful and functional products. Weavers are visionaries because they see the potential and benefit of their work even before the outcome of their efforts materializes. They have the ability to see what others cannot see. Weavers are also pragmatic. They have the skills and wherewithal to turn visions into practical realities. Weavers are sophisticated, yet often unassuming, leaders. They wish for others to focus and admire their artistic creations rather than study the mechanics of their artistry.[63]

Weavers do not just sit down and start weaving. They plan and prepare to weave. They consider the quality and availability of the materials they will use. They gather and sort the materials needed. Weavers envision what the final product might look like. Then they begin weaving to achieve a desirable outcome. But weaving is not just about practical considerations; it is also about artistry.

Artistry is particularly important to the esthetics of a weaver's finished piece. Although the weaver makes definite plans about the end product, plans often are adjusted in the actualization of their work. Weavers consequently are flexible leaders. They adjust the pattern of their pieces based on what is available, using creativity and ingenuity to alter designs as needed. As a result of their flexibility, weavers often produce better outcomes than originally intended because of their resourcefulness. A weaver weaves vision and resources into successes. Some African American breast cancer survivors function as weavers, using their available resources to create opportunities for well-being.

Felicia Knox –Weaving a Thriving Support of Faith

Felicia Knox, a thirty-something wife and mother, has a perspective on breast cancer many do not—both as a health-care professional and a survivor/thriver. Diagnosed with a Stage Two (II) breast cancer, Felicia was several months shy of reaching her two-year survivorship anniversary.[64] Like many African American women dealing with breast cancer, Felicia knew others diagnosed who later died from the disease. In fact, this had happened twice in her family. Felicia's older sisters both succumbed to breast cancer. The U.S. Preventive Services Task Force recommends that women who have first-degree family members (i.e., sisters, mother) with breast, ovarian, tubal, and peritoneal cancers should be screened for breast cancer susceptibility genes BRCA1 and BRCA2, receive genetic counseling, and then be tested for BRCA1 and BRCA2 genes.[65] Felicia has opted not to be screened, counseled, or tested.

Although Felicia never clearly indicated why she decided not to undergo BRCA1/2 testing, I suspect Felicia already knows she carries the BRCA1/2 genes. This, along with her mistrust of the current medical system she works for, one for which she believes her medical information has been used by hospital administrators against her professional advancement and to deny her requests for medical leave during her breast cancer treatment, makes it unlikely that Felicia will undergo genetic testing. Genetic testing confirming her as a BRCA1/2 carrier will further target her for discrimination. Felicia is representative of many women of color who are less likely than white women to utilize genetic services despite their increasing availability.[66] A systematic review published by Forman and Hall identified several socioeconomic barriers (i.e., time, access, language/cultural, cost) and psychosocial barriers, including medical mistrust and perceived disadvantages to genetic testing like social and insurance discrimination and social stigma, as major deterrents to Black women's being tested.[67] Felicia may have seen her sisters experience similar types of stigma and discrimination. Therefore when she was diagnosed, their experiences served as object lessons for her own breast cancer treatment decisions. Felicia chose to undergo a lumpectomy and forego adjuvant therapies against her oncologist's recommendations.

Felicia acknowledges her decision might not be right for everyone. But her biomedical knowledge and awareness of her own intolerance for treatment give her the confidence to know she is making the right decision. Therefore, at this point, she remains firm in refusing some biomedical treatments. But that does not mean Felicia is passive about her cancer treatment. No, she is aggressively intervening in her own cancer care by weaving a strategy of well-being for her cancer survivorship.

Felicia actively works to prevent cancer recurrence. She has adopted a strict vegetarian lifestyle, consuming mega doses of vitamins to boost her immune health, and tries to manage her stress to support her well-being. She consults naturopathic physicians, in addition to her regular oncology follow-ups. Felicia's approach to treating breast cancer and preventing recurrence is syncretic. She uses the best of both Western biomedicine and alternative medical treatments (i.e., naturopathy, spirituality) to meet her cancer care needs and foster well-being.

Felicia is not alone in using complementary and alternative medical (CAM) approaches for breast cancer. In addition to diet, exercise, and vitamins, Black women often include prayer, meditation, spiritual healing, and reading of scriptures as part of their CAM practices.[68] For many cancer survivors, estimated to be approximately 46 percent of those diagnosed with cancer,[69] CAM therapies (e.g., massage, yoga, meditation) are used to alleviate complications of cancer treatment, including psychosocial distress (namely, anxiety and depression), lymphedema, insomnia, fatigue and cognitive impairments. Use of CAM among breast cancer survivors is increasing and several studies have demonstrated the benefits of CAM therapies for improving cancer survivors' quality of life and managing late effects of breast cancer treatment.[70]

The reasons people with breast cancer choose CAM therapies varies, however commonly cited reasons include: negative encounters with oncologists, including perceptions of these providers as insensitive, uncaring, and harsh; fears about treatment side effects; and beliefs in the efficacy of alternative therapies.[71] Despite the benefits of many CAM therapies offer for supporting breast cancer survivors' symptom management and improved quality of life, what the effects of CAM are on breast cancer mortality are unclear.[72] Whether Felicia's reliance on CAM will increase her years of survival, particularly given her presumed genetic predisposition, remains to be seen. Yet, Felicia is willing to assume both the benefits and the burdens of choosing this complementary medical course for her treatment and disease management.

In seeking support, Felicia finds her most helpful support often comes from outside of her household. She admits that her husband does the best he can to understand what she is experiencing. But his supportive attempts have not been enough to fully meet all of her psychosocial needs. Consequently, Felicia seeks support elsewhere. She seeks support from God, her mother, her young child, co-workers, and through her active participation in church-related activities.

As a result of her cancer survivorship, Felicia feels she has been inspired by God to do more. She believes her need for support is not something she alone feels. As a result, Felicia has taken the initiative to start a breast cancer support group. She believes this is one tangible way to give and receive support from others, particularly African American breast cancer survivors. Felicia believes that hers is a mission from God.

Felicia's mission requires her to move out beyond her usual social networks to provide a space for others' support. This is part of her greater mission to bring cancer awareness to African Americans throughout her city. Achieving these goals has required Felicia to partner with other organizations, predominantly white breast cancer networks, to weave together informational and social support for African American breast cancer survivors. These were resources Felicia had not originally considered.

At first, Felicia thought these networks would be unresponsive to the specific cultural and emotional needs of African American breast cancer survivors and their communities. But Felicia's experience with breast cancer and her deepening spirituality have made her reconsider her earlier thoughts about these support networks. Felicia has adjusted her vision to weave a support network for African American breast cancer survivors. Felicia is a thriver who collaboratively weaves support for other African American breast cancer survivors' benefit. As a weaver, Felicia's leadership skills are acquired through practice. In order to effectively weave a pattern, a weaver has to know what resources are available. Felicia has assessed what psychosocial supports are available based on her own experience.

During our initial conversation, Felicia recalled her own diagnosis. She described the familial support she received. This support had not adequately met her emotional needs during her survivorship. She has seen the type of familial support she desired demonstrated elsewhere. Those experiences gave her additional perspective to evaluate the quality of support she received. These additional opportunities to witness familial support helped Felicia gauge the significance of cancer support for her well-being. Felicia spoke to these issues saying,

> When I was diagnosed I told my husband that we really needed to make sure all of our insurance and everything like that was in place. That was something we never really even focused on. And he said, "Yeah you're right." And [I asked him,]"What if it comes down to the point that I don't make it?" Because I was really more worried about my child [and his care] more than anything.
>
> He was like, "Well?" What did he say that for? It wasn't what I wanted to hear. So that's what pissed me off. And of course the tears came. And he was like, "What do you want me to do? What am I supposed to say? I don't know what to say? I can't say the right thing." And I'm like, "I don't know what you're supposed to say."

> And then he gets upset because I don't always come to him. He doesn't understand. He's like, "Why do you have to talk to them?" or "Why do you have to do this?" Not even knowing that he ain't giving me what I need. And even when I try to explain, you know, I'm probably sounding crazy.
>
> But, it's just really hard trying to explain [what I'm feeling]. I don't expect him to know and understand everything because I don't. I guess he tries the best way he can.
>
> I've found five survivors in the church and their husbands are there. [They are] right there with them, very supportive. It might be different when they get home. But, they seem real interested in what's going on. It was two men at the [church's breast cancer awareness] workshop today, which was impressive.
>
> And not just for people to see it. But, if I could just have my spouse right there with me, plugging along the way, that would be really encouraging. That's support. I think that's all in the healing [process] and all of it. So that's the biggest complaint I guess I have [about the support I receive from my husband].

The issue of social support is a paradox for Felicia and her husband. He tries to offer emotional support, but Felicia believes the support her husband provides is inadequate. When he does not offer support out of concern that he might say or do the wrong thing, Felicia believes he is being insensitive to her concerns. Felicia desires her husband's support, but is often at a loss about how to articulate the support she needs. Felicia sees the kind of familial support she would like for herself, but she is often frustrated because she cannot communicate how her husband can be supportive. Felicia's breast cancer coping abilities are complicated by these interpersonal dynamics. Consequently, Felicia relies heavily on her spirituality to adjust to cancer survivorship.

Felicia's spirituality has taught her the importance of social support for well-being. Her continuous dialogues with God have provided needed perspective about breast cancer survivorship. Felicia, as a survivor, believes that if she cannot fully receive the social support she desires, she can at least try and provide it for others.

Felicia views providing support to other African American breast cancer survivors as a divine mission. She believes serving others is the main reason God spared her life following her breast cancer diagnosis. Through her survivorship, Felicia feels compelled to offer support to other African American women undergoing and after breast cancer treatment. Felicia talked about God as being the impetus for her leadership,

> [Because of breast cancer] I have learned a whole lot. I have learned more about him [God] for one thing. I feel like that if you're paying attention to him [you'll be directed]. Because I've asked him [God], "Just show me. Use me however you want to use me. Whatever it is you're trying to do, just please use me. I'm here. Please." I beg, "Please use me."

> And I feel like part of it [is], well, I want to be able to support other Black women with cancer. Whatever the choice they decide. Wherever they are in their treatment, I want to be a resource for them on a personal level. But, at the same time I feel like he is using me as an instrument for the fact that you don't have to get chemo and radiation and still live. I truly feel like that's part of it.
>
> A lot of women don't agree with my choices. They feel like I'm just kind of being in denial. I've actually had them tell me that I'm in denial, but whatever.
>
> I truly feel like he [God] wants to set me up to be able to represent him [through cancer survivorship]. And to let people know if you trust in him, he's going to take care of you. Regardless of the outcomes, his point has been made [God will take care of you].

Through her personal experience with breast cancer, Felicia has become even more aware of public health and general public debates regarding the disease/illness of breast cancer. Many believe that her treatment decisions signal that she is in denial about having had breast cancer. Felicia disagrees.

Felicia is doing what she believes is best to effectively deal with her cancer and support her well-being. She understands that other survivors are trying to do the same. Although the roads to cancer treatment, recovery, and well-being are different, the desired outcome is the same for all women experiencing breast cancer. The goal is long-term survival following breast cancer. Whichever road a woman undergoing treatment and/or a survivor chooses, Felicia believes that their decisions should be supported. Therefore, she believes that providing helpful and nonjudgmental social support for other African American breast cancer survivors remains an important goal for her to achieve.

Not always receiving the social support she felt she needed, Felicia sought support through other social support strategies. She recalled how she came to the idea of starting her own breast cancer support group. Felicia specifically remembered the incident this way:

> [I was having] one of my sort of down periods when I was first diagnosed. And something just told me [what to do]. It was probably two or three o'clock in the morning. And the Holy Spirit said, "Just go downstairs and get on the Internet. Start searching."
>
> I didn't know what I was searching for. But, I was searching. And I came across that [the Black Women's Cancer Group website]. And I started reading it. And reading it. And the more I read, I'm like, "This sounds good." And my next thing was to try to find a local chapter because that's what I was [looking for.] I said [to myself], "I can help you. I want to be with these people." So I called them.
>
> They just kind of explained what they were all about. And I said, "Well, who [organizes the local chapter]?" Because I knew that there was a chapter here. I just knew it had to be. Somewhere in Texas it's got to be [a chapter].

> Even if I have to drive to somewhere, I know it exists. And she said, "No. It's not a chapter in Texas." So I said, "Okay Lord, it is now!"

Through communication with God (i.e., which she calls the Holy Spirit), Felicia was led to use an unlikely resource for social support. Felicia, by her own admission, is not tech savvy. Therefore, using the computer would not probably have been her primary means of seeking support or information regarding issues that were important to her. But, nevertheless, she wove its use into her support seeking.

As she searched the web, Felicia located a national African American breast cancer support group website. It was like hitting pay dirt. On this site, Felicia saw other African American women sharing the type of social support she sought. Her experience of receiving social support through the computer was empowering. The support Felicia received was so empowering, in fact, that it prompted her to want to get involved with this group. Before she even called the organization, Felicia had committed herself to working with the group and traveling, if necessary, to do so. Felicia believed being connected to this organization was necessary to her well-being.

Confident she could support other African American breast cancer survivors in this group, Felicia called the organization's headquarters. She found out that no chapter existed in the state. Instead of abandoning the idea of sharing in this group's social support, Felicia made a critical decision. She would start her own local affiliate chapter of the group.

Since that first Internet encounter, Felicia has started her own local support group. Doing so required she reach out to some unlikely partners. Felicia recalled some of her initial reservations about enlisting support for the group. She weighed these against the potential benefits of collaborating. Felicia recalled her conflicted thinking at the time,

> With that Miriam's Network [a predominantly Euro-American breast cancer awareness and advocacy organization] thing, I'm still kind of struggling with that. Because I mean, like Lord, I want us to be set apart [exclusively African American cancer survivors], but I also want us to come together [across races/ethnicities]. Because we have to come together, just humans in general, just the world. We have to somehow be able to come together, ultimately.
>
> And I feel like that I could also look at it [partnering with Miriam's Network] like he's [God] opening up this door for me now. And these people, Miriam's Network is pretty strong. I mean they could help me get what I'm trying to get. And I look at it that way.
>
> Then I try and look at it from a Black woman point of view. And it's like you weren't going there at first. What makes you think that they're going to come there just because you're there? And then I think about it and pray about it some more.
>
> And he [God] tells me, "Don't worry about that. I got that. I'll take care of that. You just do what I tell you to do." And that's where I am.

A competent weaver, Felicia assesses and reassesses the quality of the resources she is using to weave together her cancer support group. Felicia uses what Floyd-Thomas calls critical engagement,[73] a womanist ethical tenet, in considering how other African American women might perceive her support group partnering with a white cancer organization. Floyd-Thomas defines "critical engagement" as "the epistemological privilege of Black women borne of their totalistic experience with the forces of interlocking systems of oppression and strategic options they devised to undermine them."[74] Felicia understands other Black women's reticence with coming to a predominantly white cancer organization for support. She understands it because she has felt that same hesitancy about doing so.

Many Black cancer survivors are reluctant to seek social support for breast cancer in spaces and settings they consider emotionally uncomfortable to them. Their collective and individual social histories of racism, sexism, and elitism have demonstrated to them time and again that predominantly white, middle-class, and male-dominated social services (i.e., hospital-based support groups, white community–based support groups) often do not often have their best psychosocial interests at heart. Therefore, Black breast cancer survivors are reluctant to share their most intimate feelings and fears with those they do not believe equally share a commitment to their physical health and emotional well-being. Nevertheless, African American breast cancer survivors, like all breast cancer survivors, still need social support. Therefore African American breast cancer survivors often face a dilemma.

Predominantly white cancer networks often have useful support resources, but they are usually unable to persuade African American women in significant numbers to utilize them. African American survivors' past negative experiences with these networks continue to create barriers to access and use of these social supports. Therefore, more often than not, these organizations continue to remain ethnically/racially and socioeconomically homogeneous. But, Felicia is divinely inspired to believe that her support group might offer a solution to all of these issues.

Felicia does not know what the final outcome of her support group will be. But she believes her group can make a difference by bringing African American and white breast cancer survivors (across race/ethnicity, class, and gender) together in some meaningful ways. Hosting this African American breast cancer support group at Miriam's Network, Felicia believes, provides opportunities for cross-cultural dialogues around cancer survivorship. At the same time, the group provides Black cancer survivors the culturally appropriate social and informational supports many African American cancer survivors believe is important to their psychosocial cancer adjustment.

At times Felicia seems unsure about the social support network that she is weaving together. But she remains confident that God will provide her the resources needed to weave together efforts that are socially useful and culturally valuable to African American breast cancer survivors. Therefore, Felicia continues to weave a tapestry of social support for others and herself.

Felicia's abilities to weave vision and people together is something she thinks is out of character for her. This is why she believes her leadership is a divine mission. Felicia is evidencing the womanist tenet Floyd-Thomas refers to as radical subjectivity, which refers to Black women's abilities to take themselves and their subjectivity so seriously to act out of character by being bold or audacious.[75] Felicia talked about her weaving leadership in this way:

> I have never in my life dreamed of doing nothing like that [starting a support group]. I am not a people [person]. I am not just one of those outspoken [people.] Just get up. That ain't me.
>
> But at the same time, I don't have a fear about doing it either. I don't fear this because I know he's going to be there with me. He's [God] got to be. Because otherwise, I feel like I never would have initiated it, had it not been for him.
>
> Because I ain't never been a leader. Not something like this. Well of course not like this. I mean I've been an assistant radiologist. But that's not [the same thing.] That's a leader in a way. But to me this is something [else.]
>
> I have been praying that Jabez prayer. Do you know it? It's awesome. That's my life totally. It basically asks God to enlarge my territory, which means give me the opportunity [to lead].
>
> Girl, I love it! And I have prayed it. And every day I see evidence of it. Everything that I have prayed in that prayer it comes to surface every day. I've got the verse in my bathroom. I got it on my bedside table. I've got it in my car. I've got it at work. So I see it constantly. And I also see it happening in my life.

Felicia's leadership as a weaver is something completely out of character for her. She does not think of herself as a leader. Yet, she believes God sees her differently than she sees herself. As a consequence, Felicia acted boldly to organize a support group.

Felicia might not possess the personality she believes is required of a leader. Nevertheless, she has a genuine willingness to try to lead. In addition to her willingness to lead, Felicia continually relies upon her relationship with God to give her direction. Based on her "spirituality of survival," Felicia can act confidently. She is audacious because she is assured God directs and supports her leadership.

Felicia's spirituality of survival is best articulated in the prayer of Jabez she mentioned during our first encounter. The words of the prayer recorded in the Bible are as follows:

> And Jabez called on the God of Israel saying, "Oh, that You would bless me indeed, and enlarge my territory, that Your hand would be with me, and that

> You would keep me from evil that I may not cause pain!" So God granted him what he requested. (1 Chronicles 4:10) (NKJV)

Continually seeing and reciting this prayer strengthens Felicia's faith in God. Felicia's belief in God, manifested through this prayer, is based on a cultural appreciation for the nature of God's sympathetic power. God answers Jabez and makes him prosper because he earnestly asks God to do so. Because God does this for Jabez, Felicia believes God will do the same for her. Consequently Felicia believes acting similarly to Jabez will produce like responses from God through the power of *nommo*, the generative power of the spoken word.[76] By praying this prayer, Felicia believes she sets in motion God's "liberating" and sustaining power in her daily activities and leadership of the support group. This divine blessing empowers Felicia to lead. As long as she continues to believe and be led by God, then Felicia remains confident that God will continue to bless her cancer survivorship and prosper her weaving leadership.

As a weaver, Felicia's vision for the wholeness of people, particularly African American breast cancer survivors, is bigger than just the support group. Her desire is to weave her group and the social support it provides into a broader mission of health for African Americans in her city. She does this in full recognition that breast cancer support and awareness is an issue for more than just the people she knows. Felicia believes her mission to bring this message to a wider African American audience will continually require her to form partnerships with others. In attempting to reach this ultimate goal, Felicia shared the following:

> With the Miriam's thing [partnership with a white cancer support organization], you know I feel like I'm crawling. I mean before I can actually take off. Because like I told them today [some church members at a church-sponsored, health outreach activity], I don't just want to reach the people at Mt. Nebo. I mean Mt. Nebo—that's a lot of people. And that's all well and good. But we ain't the only church in the city. If I could just target five churches in the Black community [that would be worthwhile]. I would love to do [cancer outreach and provide social support to] all of them.
>
> I don't know a lot of people. If I could just hook up with people that go to other churches, that would work too. But, I don't have that kind of time to network like that. And I'm not totally trying to incorporate it at Mt. Nebo because it just can't be there. It's [awareness about African Americans and cancer] a bigger picture than that.

As Felicia's weaving abilities expand beyond the resources she possesses, she considers new partnerships to weave into the ultimate design of her cancer support group. Felicia envisions future products her group will produce. Now she works toward weaving this new vision into reality. Felicia utilizes the same leadership strategies she did in getting this cancer support group started. By forming partnerships, seeking divine guidance, and using her own creativity, Felicia continues to weave health interventions that are both helpful and meaningful for African American breast cancer survivors' well-being.

Felicia Weaving Leadership

As a weaving leader, Felicia has been endowed with a particular leadership perspective because of breast cancer. She was not receiving the support she felt she needed to adequately cope with breast cancer. This was something she felt other African American cancer survivors in her area were also missing. Rather than continue to focus only on her own situation, Felicia decided to turn the situation around. If she could not receive social support, then she would provide it to others. Felicia seeks to offer other cancer survivors social support that does not necessarily include following the dictates of biomedical regimes and treatments. Felicia works to provide nonjudgmental social support to cancer survivors. Her wish for what she would have liked more of prompted her to develop the support group.

Felicia is galvanized by a vision of providing adequate support to other African American survivors. This requires Felicia to be sensitive to other cancer survivors' needs. As a leader, Felicia is compelled to understand the ways other African American breast cancer survivors may and may not be willing to provide social support among each other and the broader community she seeks to reach. But these fears are not sufficient to deter Felicia from seeking out the maximal supports she believes Black breast cancer survivors need. Moving beyond her personal reservations, Felicia partners with others. To some, these partnerships seem unlikely and maybe even inappropriate. Felicia has become accustomed to people's doubting the soundness of her decisions at times. Despite others' reservations and her own, Felicia continues to depend on God to direct her cancer survivorship and leadership. Through these experiences, Felicia, as a weaving leader, understands it is not necessarily the materials you weave with, but the quality of the final product that is most important to promoting others' well-being.

WHAT THE "SEEKING HEALER" TEACHES ABOUT LEADERSHIP

At first glance, the story of the woman with the issue of blood, whom I call the "seeking healer" might seem out of place with other biblical heroines Porter presents as archetypes for women's leadership. Porter's leadership roles clearly situate leaders as helping others. Each of the Hebrew Bible heroines Porter bases her leadership roles on gives of themselves in service to others. They are not self-serving. However, leaders sometimes are seekers first. The seeking healer as a leadership role evidenced among some African

American breast cancer survivors falls into this category of leaders. Leaders are sometimes those who seek healing for themselves first. Their efforts to seek healing themselves become the basis out of which they help others to heal.

The seeking healer of the biblical texts (Mark 5:25–34, Matthew 9:20–22, and Luke 8:43–48) is a woman who endures a chronic disease/illness and exhausts her resources in search of a cure. All of her efforts turn out to be of no avail. This leader needs a different type of support from what she receives. Getting the support she needs requires this leader to behave in new ways. To get what she has never had (i.e., sustained health and well-being) the "seeking healer" has to do what she has never done before. The seeking healer's health-care seeking is proactive. This leader pursues unconventional approaches and unorthodox methods to support healing. The seeking healer acts in faith, believing that taking bold steps will positively affect her health.

This type of leaders has no concrete assurances that her acts will produce the desired outcomes. However, despite the uncertainty, the seeking healer remains determined to at least try. With little more to lose, a seeking healer believes she has even more to potentially gain by taking bolds steps. The seeking healer believes that achieving well-being requires womanist, radical subjectivity. Taking bold steps to reach out for support (i.e., touching Jesus's garment), the "seeking healer" attains health and well-being. By her faithful acts, the seeking healer's misfortune is transformed into triumph. The seeking healer's quality of life is also transformed. This leader knows she has been healed. Yet, the seeking healer is often content to remain anonymous. Sufficiently thankful to be healed, the seeking healer does not search out an opportunity to publicly share her experiences. Instead, this type of leader has to be challenged to speak. The seeking healer speaks because the circumstances dictate that she must.

When the seeking healer, as leader, shares her story, she does it to save herself. It is not what others have done or attempted to do for this woman's health that is most important. The seeking healer's courageous acts (i.e., reaching out for support, telling her story), coupled with her abiding faith, are what are most efficacious to her healing. The seeking healer determines her own positive health outcome by searching for healing. As a leader, the seeking healer by her actions realizes she possesses the power to heal. The ability to provide helpful support is an attribute seeking healers as leaders often find surprising about themselves. The seeking healer is an effective leader because of her humility. But nevertheless, the seeking healer is a reluctant leader because she continually underestimates her own leadership abilities.

Hilda Holmes—Thriver as Seeking Healer

Hilda Holmes, a fifty-three-year-old administrator, is a twelve-year breast cancer survivor.[77] She was diagnosed with breast cancer first at age forty. Following her fortieth birthday, within the span of a few short weeks, she underwent a mastectomy, with no additional adjuvant therapy recommended. Two years later, Hilda had a breast cancer recurrence. This time, Hilda underwent a mastectomy to remove her remaining breast. Several years following her second surgery, Hilda had reconstructive surgery performed to replace her removed breasts. Complications from reconstructive surgery made Hilda's recovery painful both physically and emotionally. She is often reluctant to share this painful experience with other women contemplating having reconstruction. Hilda does not want to frighten other women any more than they already are as a result of breast cancer.

Growing up as an asthmatic child, Hilda often felt as if her condition set her socially apart from others. Her condition stigmatized her further by making her feel like she was not useful to her family or others. Not being able to participate in many of the activities other children did, Hilda thought of herself as physically weak and emotionally fragile. These feelings helped to foster her shy and introverted nature.

Hilda did not try things she thought beyond her abilities because she thought she would fail. The psychosocial pain she felt often made Hilda want to give up and die because it did not seem that circumstances would ever get better. Hilda continued to feel this way for much of her adult life. Content to allow others to take care of her and make decisions for how she should act and respond, Hilda repeated the same patterns as an adult she had as a child. When she was diagnosed with breast cancer, she followed the medical advice her physicians gave and relied on her family's emotional support to cope with her treatment and recovery. After surgery, Hilda confined herself to her home for several weeks because she was ashamed that she had had breast cancer. As she had when she was a child, she believed others would treat her differently. Hilda's breast cancer recurrence, however, changed everything for her.

When Hilda was diagnosed with breast cancer for the second time, she reached a point where she had had enough. She was ready to fight for her life. Hilda made a conscious decision to fight to survive and thrive beyond breast cancer. Hilda would proactively take charge of her well-being. Hilda's resolve was tested more than once, but she remained determined to press forward until her change came. Although Hilda currently sees her experience with breast cancer as a tragedy, she believes there is an even greater tragedy than this. For her an even greater tragedy is to say nothing about her breast cancer experience and to not offer support to those most in need. Hilda understands these tragedies because she has experienced both.

When her cousin was diagnosed with terminal cancer, Hilda fell silent. She had had both of her surgeries by then. She was successfully surviving breast cancer. Yet Hilda's cousin's dying represented her worst fear materialized, her own death. Hilda did not know what to say or how to support her cousin's dying. So Hilda avoided her cousin. Hilda's fear of death had made her mute. And then before Hilda could gather up sufficient courage to provide support, her cousin died. Hilda grieved her cousin's death and felt ashamed because of it. Hilda thought about opportunities she felt she had missed to support her cousin. She felt deep remorse because her fears had prevented her from supporting someone she really cared about. These feelings would not go away even after she sought forgiveness for them.

Hilda needed to find a way to make up for the support she had been unable to give her cousin. Hilda wanted to act in a way that honored her cousin's memory. Most importantly, Hilda needed her own emotional release for the feelings of shame burdening her. But acting would necessitate Hilda's giving more of herself than she usually was comfortable doing. Hilda would have to behave in new ways to achieve the emotional catharsis necessary for her well-being.

It was with her cousin's death that Hilda started speaking to other breast cancer survivors. Telling her story of survivorship is her way of alleviating the emotional distress she felt following her cousin's death. At the same time Hilda uses this strategy to find the support she needs, sharing her testimony also helps others. Hilda's testimony gives other breast cancer survivors hope about their own continued survivorship.

Hilda does not actively seek out opportunities to tell her story. Nevertheless when she is presented with the opportunity, she tells her story. She uses these situations to tell others, particularly those who have not had breast cancer, what it means to have the disease and explains cancer survivorship. She has spoken publicly about her cancer experience to professional and community audiences. Hilda often starts off relaying her testimony rather timidly. But as she continues to share her story she increasingly becomes more confident in talking about her cancer survivorship.

Breast cancer has also prompted Hilda to rekindle her artistic abilities. She produces visual images of what healing, survivorship, and thriving are about. Hilda started taking photographs as a survival strategy to aid her personal psychosocial adjustment and well-being. By taking pictures of scenes from nature, Hilda is often reminded, through the images she sees, of God's presence around her. Beyond helping her adjustment during her cancer survivorship, these photographs have helped her resolve many personal issues including the grief she experienced as a result of her mother's death. The photographs Hilda takes help heal her.

Since taking up photography again, Hilda has shared these pictures and testimonies with others. Many people tell her how helpful her pictures and words are to their healing. Hilda is continually amazed by others' affirmation of her visual artistry. Hilda takes pictures to save her life. Pictures are a way of telling her survivorship story. Yet others also find healing and inspiration from these same images and what they convey.

Hilda, through her experience with breast cancer, has come full circle. She seeks opportunities to care for herself and others. Although at times she still fears recurrence, Hilda continually seeks new strategies to give her peace of mind. Hilda pursues these new strategies to maintain her emotional adjustment and stability. She uses these strategies to attain a better quality of life and promote personal well-being. She seeks and finds new ways to heal herself, from the inside out. In turn, Hilda also possesses the ability to heal.

At the same time Hilda knows that her actions have changed her, at times she still sees herself as the ineffective, timid, sickly girl she felt she was growing up. Although Hilda is thankful for her cancer survivorship, she is intentionally unassuming. She would have been comfortable, by her own admission, living out her survivorship in virtual anonymity. But, the memory of her cousin's death makes it impossible for Hilda to live in the shadows. So she vocalizes her leadership when she is called upon to do so. Admittedly, Hilda does this more often to help herself.

Yet, when Hilda acts as a seeking healer, she is often surprised when people tell her how her leadership helped them heal. Hilda sees these acts merely as helpful to herself. She rarely thinks of her leadership as providing support and hope to others. In fact, she is often concerned that others might reject her leadership or perceive it to be a nuisance. Hilda's story and her leadership are both indicative of a seeking healer experience.

The seeking healer of the New Testament accounts is at first a tragic figure. She is a woman who has a disease/illness for which her community stigmatizes her. Because of the fear of social rejection, the seeking healer does not share her condition with many, instead shouldering the illness burden by herself. The seeking healer feels ashamed because of her condition and is also made to feel ashamed by others because of it. The seeking healer's tragedy is one she is compelled to shield from others.

The same is true for Hilda. Being diagnosed with breast cancer is a tragedy for Hilda. She was so frightened by her first diagnosis and treatment that for the longest time she would not even say the word "cancer." Instead, Hilda veiled her condition by not telling people that she had had a mastectomy and opting to have reconstructive surgery.

She did this because she was afraid others might treat her differently (i.e., stigmatize her) or reject her because she had breast cancer. Breast cancer was a condition that made Hilda ashamed to share publicly. Hilda discussed her initial feelings about having breast cancer this way:

> In the beginning I thought it was a tragedy. Well [because] it was cancer. And just the word cancer scares you. And I had seen people with cancer before.
>
> He [physician] actually didn't say "cancer" he just said, "Malignant. Malignant." The other doctor [oncologist] was the one that said, "Cancer." And it was like I really didn't want to hear that word. Just don't say the word.
>
> And I didn't say it for a long time. It was just frightening to hear that you have cancer. And for a long time I had a hard time saying, "I had breast cancer." I would always say, "I had to have a mastectomy," not thinking that [if] you have a mastectomy, usually it's for cancer. But yeah, for a while there I thought it was a tragedy. But, it got better. Everything gets better with time.

At first breast cancer seemed like a tragedy to Hilda. The word "cancer" and what it might mean for her physical and psychosocial health were frightening to her. Hilda's survivorship after her initial diagnosis was not easy. At first she felt ashamed because of her cancer. Then she was afraid that others would socially reject her. Her fears of death created additional stress. Breast cancer, especially the first time around, seemed as if it might be a tragedy forever. But, somewhere in Hilda's mind remained a hope that things might eventually get better.

Initially, in the interview, Hilda did not identify the exact thing that prompted her to change her mind about breast cancer. Her cousin's death and its emotional impact were revealed in a later discussion. Hilda's cousin's death in many ways was a catalyst that motivated Hilda to work to make her survivorship better, especially the second time around. In the biblical accounts of the woman who sought healing, what motivated her to seek healing differently is not recorded. All that is recorded is what she did. And because of what the seeking healer and Hilda did, their situations "got better."

But before either the seeking healer or Hilda even thought of things getting better, they had suffered for many years being chronically ill. As a result, of their chronic conditions, they both relied on other's support. For Hilda, this made her feel inadequate and helpless. The emotional and physical fatigue caused by Hilda's asthma as a child often made her want to give up and die. This might have been how the seeking healer experiencing the chronicity of her debilitating condition might has felt as well. Hilda shared her feelings about growing up with asthma:

> I grew up with asthma. And so I stayed sick a lot and I gave up a lot, you know. Whenever I had an asthma attack I would just fall apart and my mother would have to rush me to the hospital. And I used to, you know, just want to die because I was tired of being sick all the time. And then when they told me I had cancer, instead of wanting to die, I was ready to fight. [As a result of having breast cancer] I learned that I was stronger than I gave myself credit for.
>
> It made me be more [assertive], you know—trust in myself, you know. Give myself credit for fighting, you know. I was like my mother. You know, I

> was fighting back. And so it gave me courage; made my faith stronger. I'm a better person for that.

Hilda, like the seeking healer, had perhaps in some ways grown accustomed to being ill. They both would seek treatment to alleviate their symptoms, but they never were able to find a cure. Fatigue became a constant companion to both. Hilda came to accept illness as a part of life.

With Hilda's initial diagnosis and treatment, she came to think of breast cancer in the same way she did asthma. Breast cancer, like asthma, brought shame and feelings of worthlessness. Both even brought what biomedicine might label as chronic depression. Hilda thought that cancer would forever be a part of her life, something to be tolerated and managed. Hilda did what her physicians told her to do and she existed with the disease/illness. The same would probably have been the case for the biblical character from whom the seeking healer archetype is derived.

With her breast cancer recurrence, Hilda finally decided she had had enough. Hilda was, in the immortal words of the civil rights activist Fannie Lou Hamer, "sick and tired of being sick and tired."[78] Enough was enough. For Hilda and the seeking healer, there had to be something better than just surviving. Hilda's struggle against her pain transformed her into a change agent. Hilda became more determined than ever to fight to live. In order to live, Hilda had to think and behave differently.

Although, by having breast cancer, Hilda found a new determination to fight and challenge the disease, the defeats of her past at times resurfaced. She thought about what if she failed to receive the support she needed to live? Why even try. Hilda had to learn to undo those kinds of patterns. As Hilda reflected on things she has learned having had breast cancer, she shared,

> [When I told other people about having breast cancer] I didn't feel comfortable, at first. I meet some people at work who went through the same thing and we would talk about it. And afterwards, you know, I think we felt better.

At first, Hilda as a seeking healer, feared disclosing her identity as a breast cancer survivor. She believed that others might treat her differently. Consequently, she took small steps as a leader. She would share her breast cancer experience with a few people. Sharing her experience made her feel better for a while. Yet, her relief was short-lived. What Hilda wanted was an experience that would revolutionize her survivorship indefinitely. Seeking healers' being prompted to finally act and speak is brought to bear by circumstances that will not be addressed in any other way. They are tired of living the way they have been living. They fear dying. Therefore, some major situation has to change the way they view themselves. As a result, of this event, they will move from being reactive to being proactive. Hilda recalled the circumstances of breast cancer that caused her to change the way she viewed her cancer survivorship and her subsequent leadership. She shared the following:

> I don't normally talk to people that much, but my cousin, one of my cousins, died from breast cancer. She was thirty-four. And it was after she died [that I started sharing my experience]. Before she died I had a hard time talking to her. And I felt really bad about it. The reason I had a hard time was because I knew she was dying. And I knew that I had had breast cancer and I came through it. And I didn't know how to relate to her, to her dying.
>
> So after she died I told her mother. I said, "I'm sorry I couldn't be with her like I should have been." She said, "Pearl knew that." She said, "Every day Pearl would ask about you. Wanted to know, make sure that you were okay." And I felt really bad that I didn't see her like I should have.
>
> I thought. Then I said, "I'm going to have to do better. I'm going to have to start opening up to people." I said, "I should have opened up to her." And to this day I feel very bad about that. But her mother sort of helped me through it. She said, "She understood and Pearl understood."

Hilda's cousin's death served as a major turning point in Hilda's survivorship. Although she successfully came through both of her surgeries, fear of death paralyzed Hilda. She feared acknowledging what had happened to her. Hilda did not know what to say to her cousin as she was dying. Even after her cousin's death, the memory of her own inability to support her cousin still haunted Hilda.

Hilda sought relief from her distress after her cousin's death. Her cousin's mother told her that her cousin understood she was too frightened to speak. She even told Hilda that instead of being angry, her cousin had been concerned about Hilda's emotional well-being. The memory of missed opportunities haunts Hilda. The only way to address it is for Hilda to speak up and share her story with others. She does this to save herself.

Hilda's speaking her truth helps relieve the angst she feels about her cousin's death. Hilda talks about what her cousin's death means to her. She also discusses how this circumstance affects her own seeking healer leadership. Hilda shares what her thoughts were following her cousin's death:

> So after that [my cousin's death] when I know of someone who has [cancer], who is going through what I went through, I let them know that they can get through [cancer]. You know [they can still be hopeful] even if their cancer has progressed to a [terminal] point. It's like one lady told me, "Looking at you gives me hope."
>
> [Sharing my story] took a while. Sometimes I still don't open up like I should. I'm trying to do better. I'm trying to get more involved in the breast cancer research and talking to people. I've even thought about being a volunteer. But, I haven't gotten to that point.

> [Through breast cancer and my cousin's death] I see people in a different light too. You know, I see people and I want to be able to help them. I've always wanted to help them. But, you know how you sit back and say, "Somebody else is going to do it." So I had to learn to undo that in my past. So I have more tolerance of things now because I had to be helped. So it makes you stronger.

The seeking healer's actions are often enacted for their emotional benefit. They need comfort and reassurance that things will be okay. So they seek out opportunities to receive support. The seeking healer necessarily does this in ways often outside of their typical behavior patterns. In seemingly unconventional ways, seeking healers receive the support they are looking for. Unbeknown to them, they also provide support to others. The fact that seeking healers are able to help someone else with their story continually surprises them. The same remains true for Hilda.

Hilda shares her experiences with other survivors as a way of seeking her own psychosocial support. It is her way of atoning for past failures. These experiences help Hilda to heal emotionally. Because of Hilda's past and her introverted nature, she is not usually given to speak up or share her feelings with others. She readily admits that this is a part of her leadership she continually works on. There are some situations (e.g., volunteering, participating in clinical trials, etc.) Hilda still does not feel comfortable participating in. But that does not mean she does not consider these as options for the future. At the present, she exercises her leadership in those situations that bring her the most immediate psychosocial reward.

Hilda also talked about her personality and how that has been affected by breast cancer. She describes some additional situations in which she has used her seeking leadership. Hilda attempts to reach out to help herself cope by receiving support from other cancer survivors. In the process of their sharing, Hilda gives other women hope about their own survivorship. Their responses to her support are overwhelmingly positive.

This was not the response Hilda expected. She used to worry that she was being a nuisance to other survivors with her telephone calls. But she came to find out that these survivors perceive Hilda differently than she perceives herself. They see her support as vital to their well-being. She helps them more effectively cope and adjust to the circumstances breast cancer brings into their lives. Hilda seeks support, but simultaneously she provides psychosocial healing to others and to herself. Hilda described her seeking healer leadership this way:

> No. I've never been an outward person. That's the way I've always been. But having cancer—it brings out a lot in you. You just want to let people know that you can survive. And I know everybody doesn't survive, but some people do. And even the ones who are going through it [need to] know this.

> I had another close friend who died from it. And we talked every day. But, I didn't realize how sick she was until later because hers came back. And then a few months later she passed away. And I felt that we gave each other hope.
>
> I have another friend in New Jersey and we talk back and forth. She's got ovarian cancer. I talked to her one night and she said, "Just talking to you," she said, "we pick each other up." So that made me feel good because I thought I was bothering her, you know. And she was telling me that [about my] call[ing] to check on her. She said, "When I hear your voice," she said, "I feel better." That made me feel pretty good.
>
> And just the thought that I'm opening up to people and helping people, it gives me more strength. It just helps to talk to people. It releases some of the fear I have when I talk about it. And it's like I'm "useful." I use that word all the time. I guess you must think that I have always felt I wasn't useful or something. But it is when I can see it in people that they have hope [that is when I know I have been useful]. You know you've gone twelve or thirteen years free, they say, "Well maybe this can happen to us." And so that's what helps me.

The seeking healer in the biblical text came looking for a healing miracle for herself. What she found in the process was that the very thing she came looking for, she already possessed. The seeking healer, by her faithful and determined leadership, possessed the keys to bring about and sustain her own healing. Hilda never thought that she could positively affect her health in this way. She had always relied on others to help her cope. She had also adjusted to being chronically sick. Now, with a particularly dramatic event, her life was transformed.

Hilda's cousin's death was as a watershed moment. She could no longer sit back and let others handle the situation or provide support to those in need. Hilda learned to do this, even though she was afraid. However, even her fear was not longer sufficient to keep her silent. Hilda survived breast cancer and, with her cousin's death, now she is challenged to share her testimony with others. Hilda can no longer remain quiet about surviving cancer; she has to tell others. The memories of her cousin's death and her own inability to provide support to her cousin as she was dying will not let Hilda remain mute. As a seeking healer, Hilda continues to speak.

Hilda as a Seeking Healer

Hilda evidences qualities inherent to the seeking healer. Limited by her physical conditions, this leader often develops a sense of self, which continually makes them feel inadequate. They believe that others must continually do for them because they are unable to do for themselves. This is how Hilda saw herself. That was until breast cancer.

Breast cancer changed the way Hilda sees herself. She can no longer be passive about her breast cancer survivorship. In order to live, Hilda has become active in her well-being as she never had before. She has learned to endure whatever potential risks exist (e.g., social rejection) in order to achieve health and well-being. As Hilda recognizes, ingrained behavioral patterns are often hard to change. It was not until she experienced a particularly pivotal life event that Hilda's self-defeating and self-effacing behaviors could no longer suffice.

The death of Hilda's cousin and her own need for support challenge her to speak. She has to tell others of her survivorship. Hilda was at first doing this not so much for the listener's benefit, but more for her own. In telling her story, Hilda exerts leadership necessary to insure her own emotional healing. In telling her story, Hilda came to discover that what she is seeking, interestingly enough, she is also providing. Hilda learned to heal others by telling her story and heal herself at the same time.

Hilda's story gives others hope. They are receptive to her message, even when she thinks they might feel otherwise. Peoples' receptivity to her story and the pictures she takes empower her and give her emotional strength, which continue to help her survive and thrive. Hilda as a seeking healer brings healing to others as she heals herself.

THRIVING ROLES AS A BREAST CANCER SURVIVORSHIP EPISTEMOLOGY

For some African American breast cancer survivors, the thriving roles described here are located in Christianity, a familiar religious cultural tradition. As a consequence, embedded in these leadership roles are Christian values and beliefs (e.g., faith in God, reliance on the Holy Spirit for direction) that resonate with how these cancer survivors see the world. As part of womanist theology, the use of biblical texts and female biblical actors as resources for making sense of the world and operating in it are not uncommon for Black women.[79] The values female biblical figures display help many African American breast cancer survivors understand who they are. As well, these female biblical actors and their values influence Black women's agency and leadership. African American cancer survivors' theology serves as an important cultural vehicle to understand their thoughts and actions. These beliefs, along with their experiences as African American women, inform an epistemology of the African American breast cancer experience.

The roles described here demonstrate that African American breast cancer survivors actively use their experiences with breast cancer to beneficially affect the lives of others. As is indicative of women's leadership, Black women exhibit an ethic of care[80] that prompts them to become bridge leaders who link needs and consciousness with organizations and resources that support Black people's survival.[81] These African American thriving leaders use their differing abilities to provide hope, comfort, and voice to those affected by breast cancer. These survivors' efforts also change their perspectives on cancer. Instead of focusing on the negatives, these African American cancer survivors focus on the cultural and social benefits of their survivorship as ways to exercise leadership. These survivors use their cultural and social histories as African American women to affect positive health outcomes and promote well-being for themselves and others with breast cancer.

These African American breast cancer survivors as leaders use their resources (e.g., social networks, stories) to promote positive social change in their communities by becoming "caretakers of the race."[82] Indicative of Black female leadership, these Black cancer survivors exemplify survival techniques (e.g., support seeking) that demonstrate their creativity and commitment for group well-being.[83] Like African American foremothers before them, their efforts often remain invisible to the general and academic public. Nevertheless they and other women they represent use varied forms of Black women's leadership borne out of a "culture of political resistance"[84] against race, gender, and class oppression to nurture well-being from the inside out. Theirs are stories of struggle and the ongoing search for well-being, for themselves and others. Theirs are not just survivor stories. They are Black breast cancer thriver stories of leadership and well-being.

NOTES

1. Townes, Emilie. (1993). "Living in the New Jerusalem: The Rhetoric and Movement of Liberation in the House of Evil." In *A Troubling in My Soul: Womanist Perspectives on Evil & Suffering*, 78–91. Maryknoll, NY: Orbis Books, 84.
2. Porter, J. (2000). *Leading Ladies: Transformative Biblical Images of Women's Leadership*. Philadelphia: Innisfree Press.
3. Neufeldt V., and Guarlnik D. (Eds.). (1998). *Webster's New World College Dictionary*, 3rd ed. New York: Simon & Schuster.
4. I first became acquainted with the term "thriver" during the eighth Biennial Intercultural Cancer Council Meeting in Washington, D.C. (February 2001). The anthropologist Susan Shinagawa used the term to describe herself. A cancer "thriver" thrives despite the disease and uses their experience to make a difference for others. Once a survivor does this, then they are a thriver and not just a survivor. I found this construct to be helpful in conceptualizing breast cancer survivors' agency.
5. Rosser-Mims, D. (2010). "Black Feminism: An Epistemological Framework for Exploring How Race and Gender Impact Black Women's Leadership Development." *Advancing Women in Leadership Journal*, *30* (15): 1–10.
6. Vetter, L. (2010). "Overview: Feminist Theories of Leadership. In K. O'Connor (Ed.), *Gender and Women's Leadership: A Reference Handbook*, vol. 1, 3–10. Thousand Oaks, CA: SAGE Publications.
7. Ibid., 1.
8. Ibid.
9. Locke, J. (1989). *The Second Treatise on Civil Government.* Amherst, MA: Prometheus Books.
10. Ibid.
11. Vetter. "Overview," 5.
12. Ibid.

13. Rousseau, J.-J. (1985). *The Government of Poland.* (W. Kendall, Trans.) Indianapolis: Hackett.

14. Rousseau, J.-J. (1987). *Basic Political Writings.* (D. Cress, Trans.) Indianapolis: Hackett.

15. Vetter. "Overview," 5.

16. Rousseau, *Basic Political Writings*.

17. Vetter. "Overview," 6.

18. Ibid.

19. Foucault, M. (1980) in C. Gordon (Ed.), *Power/Knowledge: Selected Interviews and Other Writings, 1972–1977.* New York: Pantheon Books.

20. Foucault, M. (1995). *Discipline & Punish: The Birth of the Prison.* (A. Sheridan, Trans.) New York: Random House.

21. Vetter. "Overview," 6.

22. Tronto, J. (1993). *Moral Boundaries: A Political Argument for an Ethic of Care.* New York: Routledge.

23. Ibid.

24. Pittinsky, T., Bacon, L., and Welle, B. (2007). "The Great Women Theory of Leadership? Perils of Positive Streotypes and Precarious Pedestals." In B. Kellerman, and D. Rhode (Eds.), *Women and Leadership: The State of Play and Strategies for Change,* 93–127. San Francisco: Jossey-Bass.

25. Ibid., 96.

26. Vetter. "Overview," 8.

27. Caruso, D., Mayer, J., and Salovey, P. (2002). "Emotional Intelligence and Emotional Leadership." In R. Riggio, S. Murphy, and F. Pirozzolo (Eds.), *Multiple Intelligences and Leadership*, 55–74. Mahwah, NJ: Lawrence Erlbaum.

28. Vetter. "Overview," 8.

29. Ibid., 8.

30. Young, M. (2000). *Inclusion and Democracy*. New York: Oxford University Press.

31. Ibid.

32. Ibid.

33. Ibid.

34. hooks, b. (2000). *Feminist Theory: From Margin to Center,* 2nd ed. Cambridge, MA: South End Press.

35. Collins, P. H. (2000). *Black Feminist Thought: Knowledge, Consciousness, and the Politics of Empowerment.* New York: New York University Press.

36. Ibid.

37. Rosser-Mims, "Black Feminism," 7.

38. Crenshaw, K. (1989). "Demarginalizing the Intersection of Race and Sex: A Black Feminist Critique of Antidiscrimination Doctrine, Feminist Theory and Antiracist Politics." *University of Chicago Legal Forum*, 139–167.

39. Smooth, W. (2010). "Intersectionalities of Race and Gender and Leadership." In O'Connor, *Gender and Women's Leadership*, 34.

40. Ibid., 35.

41. Robnett, B. (1997). *How Long? How Long? African American Women and the Struggle for Civil Rights.* New York: Oxford University Press.

42. Collins. *Black Feminist Thought*, 11.

43. Robnett, B. (2010). "Women Leaders in the Civil Rights Movement." In O'Connor, *Gender and Women's Leadership*, 196–203.

44. Ibid., 196.

45. Deckman, M. (2010). "Women as Leaders in Protestant Denominations." In O'Connor, *Gender and Women's Leadership*, 549.

46. Gilkes, C. (2001). *If It Wasn't for the Women: Black Women's Experience and Womanist Culture in Church and Community.* Maryknoll, NY: Orbis Books.

47. Weems, R. (1989). *Just a Sister Away: Understanding the Timeless Connection Between Women of Today and Women in the Bible.* New York: Warner.

48. Grant, J. (1989). *White Women's Christ and Black Women's Jesus: Feminist Christology and Womanist Response.* Atlanta: Scholars Press; and Williams, D. (1993). *Sisters in the Wilderness: The Challenge of Womanist God-talk.* Maryknoll, NY: Orbis Books.
49. Ibid., 26.
50. Ibid.
51. Brown-Douglass, K. D. (1993). "Womanist Theology: What Is Its Relationship to Black Theology?" In J. H. Cone and G. S. Wilmore (Eds.), *Black Theology: A Documentary History*, vol. 2, *1980–1992*, 290–299. Maryknoll, NY: Orbis Books.
52. Deckman, "Women as Leaders," 550.
53. Tronto. *Moral Boundaries*.
54. Porter, *Leading Ladies*.
55. Walker, A. (1993). "In Search of Our Mothers' Gardens." In J. H. Cone and G. S. Wilmore (Eds.), *Black Theology: A Documentary History*, vol. 1, *1960–1979*. Maryknoll, NY: Orbis Books
56. Floyd-Thomas, S. (2006). *Deeper Shades of Purple.* New York: NYU Press.
57. Porter, *Leading Ladies*, 15.
58. Burns, J. M. (1978). *Leadership.* New York: Harper & Row Publishing.
59. Bennis, W., and Nanus, B. (1997). *Leaders: Strategies for Taking Charge.* Second Edition. New York: Harper & Row Publishing.
60. Floyd-Thomas, S. (2017, April 19). Womanist Ethical Language Handout.
61. Ibid.
62. Taylor, E. J. (2000). "Transformation of Tragedy among Women Surviving Breast Cancer." *Oncology Nursing Forum*, *27* (5): 781–788.
63. Porter, *Leading Ladies*, 15.
64. Felicia Knox is a pseudonym and personal details of her life have been fictionalized.
65. Moyer, V., and U.S. Preventive Services Task Force. (2014). "Risk Assessment, Genetic Counseling, and Genetic Testing for BRCA-Related Cancers in Women: U.S. Preventive Services Task Force Recommendations Statement." *Annals of Internal Medicine*, *160* (4): 271–281.
66. Halbert, C., Kessler, L., Troxel, A., Stopfer, J., and Domcheck, S. (2010). "Effects of Genetic Counseling and Testing for BRCA1 and BRCA2 Mutations in African American Women: A Randomized Trial." *Public Health Genomics*, *13*, 440–448; and Armstrong, K., Micco, E., Carney, A., Stopfer, J., and Putt, M. (2005). "Racial Differences in the Use of BRCA1/2 Testing among Women with a Family History of Breast or Ovarian Cancer." *JAMA*, *293*, 1729–1736.
67. Forman, A., and Hall, M. (2009). "Influence of Race/Ethncity on Genetic Counseling and Testing for Hereditary Breast and Ovarian Cancer." *The Breast Journal*, *15* (s1): 56–62; and Sheppard, V., Mays, D., LaVeist, T., and Tercyak, K. (2013). "Medical Mistrust and Self-Efficacy Influence Black Women's Level of Engagement in BRCA1/2 Genetic Counseling and Testing." *Journal of the National Medical Association*, *105* (1): 17–22.
68. Lambe, C. (2013). "Complementary and Alternative Therapy Use in Breast Cancer: Notable Findings." *Journal of Christian Nursing*, *30* (4): 219–225.
69. Horneber, M., Bueschel, G., Dennert, G., Less, D., Ritter, E., and Zwahlen, M. (2012). "How Many Cancer Patients Use Complementary and Alternative Medicine: A Systematic Review and Metaanalysis." *Integrative Cancer Therapies*, *11*, 187–203.
70. Blaes, A., Kreitzer, M., Torkelson, C., and Haddad, T. (2011). "Nonpharmacologic Complementary Therapies in Symptom Management for Breast Cancer Survivors." *Seminars in Oncology*, *38*, 394–402; and Henneghan, A., and Harrison, T. (2015). "Complementary and Alternative Medicine Therapies as Symptom Management Strategies for the Late Effects of Breast Cancer Treatment." *Journal of Holistic Nursing*, *33* (1): 84–97.
71. Citrin, D., Bloom, D., Grutsch, J., Mortensen, S., and Lis, C. (2012). "Beliefs and Perceptions of Women with Newly Diagnosed Breast Cancer Who Refused Conventional Treatment in Favor of Alternative Therapies." *The Oncologist*, *17*, 607–612.
72. Neuhouser, M., et al. (2016). "Use of Complementary and Alternative Medicine and Breast Cancer Survival in the Health, Eating, Activity and Lifestyle Study." *Breast Cancer Research and Treatment*, *160*, 539–546.

73. Floyd-Thomas. *Deeper Shades of Purple.*
74. Ibid.
75. Ibid.
76. Jackson, R., and Richardson, E. (Eds.). (2003). *Understanding African American Rhertoric: Classical and Contemporary Innovations.* New York: Routledge.
77. Hilda Holmes is a pseudonym and personal details of her life have been fictionalized.
78. Lee, C. K. (1999). *For Freedom's Sake: The Life of Fannie Lou Hamer*. Urbana: University of Illinois Press.
79. Weems. *Just a Sister Away*.
80. Tronto. *Moral Boundaries*.
81. Robnett. "Women Leaders in the Civil Rights Movement."
82. Collins. *Black Feminist Thought.*
83. Rosser-Mims, "Black Feminism," 7.
84. Collins, *Black Feminist Thought*.

Chapter Six

Black Cancer Survivors' Transformative Theology of Hope

"Cancer doesn't discriminate. It doesn't care who you are. It doesn't care whether or not you are ready." That is what Constance, an African American breast cancer survivor, once told a group of survivors.[1] Yet, while breast cancer affects women and men of diverse backgrounds, it disproportionately affects some populations more than others. While white women are diagnosed with breast cancer more than other ethnic groups, African American women, when diagnosed with breast cancer, succumb at a higher rate.[2] As well, aggressive and more lethal forms of breast cancer are more often diagnosed among younger African American women, especially those under forty-five years of age.[3] Saying that breast cancer is an equal opportunity menace belies the reality of the disease. It is a disease that does not play fair.

For those diagnosed with breast cancer, particularly African American women for whom the statistical odds of survival are shortest and others, hope is an important resource.[4] Hope is what these African American survivors hold on to when their bodies, support systems, and even biomedicine fail them. Hope is the fuel of their Christian theology. It is located in a transcendent God, the one they talk to when they cannot talk to anyone else. Their theology affirms that the triune God sees and identifies with them, co-sufferers with them, and is a God who can liberate them from their suffering.[5] God functions for Black breast cancer survivors as their secure base and safe haven, a close attachment relationship to which these Black women turn in times of distress for comfort.[6] Black breast cancer survivors' *hope in God* is also transformational. This hope is grounded in their *faith in God*, the one who can transform people and situations, ever turning what is seemingly negative for a greater good.[7] Hope even in the face of seeming hopelessness is what many African American women with cancer draw upon for strength and to sustain their faith.

Many African American survivors understand breast cancer through the cultural lens of their Christian faith. They understand breast cancer as a type of trouble in which God intervenes and prevails. Their theology underscores that God intervenes, sustains and triumphs over troubles. Black women with breast cancer know this God in their troubles. Theirs is a God who has never failed them yet. Additionally, they situate their faith in their individual and collective experiences as Black women for whom the intersections of racism, class, and sexism impact their health. They know God in the midst of these troubles too. As Jones terms it, these breast cancer survivors are "inside experts," who theorize Black women's oppression and understand Christian theology from the inside out.[8] As "inside experts" and everyday theologians, these survivors theorize, ask theological questions, and seek answers in the context of their lived experiences and narratives.

Out of this, Black women affected by breast cancer construct a cultural theology of well-being. This theology stems from hope born out of "visionary pragmatism" as Collins calls it, a hope that believes in and assumes the best that is possible, while simultaneously pays attention to the current circumstances and works toward its achievement in the present. Black women's theology of well-being believes in a transcendent, yet ever-present triune God who intercedes to mediate the troubles of breast cancer for Black women.[9] This God is one who sees and co-labors with the oppressed and walks with Black women through the *valley of the shadow of death* that breast cancer brings and is *grace and mercy that follows them all the days of their lives* before, during, and after breast cancer treatment.[10] This is the practical theology African American breast cancer survivors share among themselves and with others. These Black cancer survivors nurture their theology of well-being by talking to God and others. This God talk gives them resources to prevail against breast cancer.

Emile Durkheim, in his interpretation of religion, points out that religion is meaningful to its adherents for two reasons—namely, that it provides truths and strength. As he says,

> The believer who has communicated with his [or her] god is not merely a man [or woman] who sees new truths of which the unbeliever is ignorant; he [or she] is a man [or woman] who is *stronger*. He [or she] feels within him [or her] more force, either to endure the trials of existence, or to conquer them.[11]

Black women with breast cancer indeed acquire new truths through their God talk. The truth they acquire is that they can survive even in the face of the profound menace breast cancer is to Black women. The new truth revealed to them is that death is not something to fear, nor is suffering what

God intends for them. The new truth they gain from their God talk is that God walks with, struggles with/for them, and will keep them through it all. These are some of the new truths Black women see through their God talk.

Black women with breast cancer, further agreeing with Durkheim, would also argue that they gain strength from God. Talking to God helps them not to panic when they are diagnosed and gives them resolve to endure treatment. Their God talk gives them strength to let down their guard as Strong Black women, risk being seen as vulnerable, seek help, and struggle against depression and pain. God also helps them to regain their equilibrium. Yet, God talk does more than this. God talk gives them the strength to conquer the trials of breast cancer, helping them to forge new ways of being. In conquering their fears, these Black women become change agents they never knew themselves to be. Equipped with God-given strength, these Black breast cancer survivors push through breast cancer to become change agents who, as Black women leaders, use their experiences, resources, and creativity to forge healing for themselves and others. Yes, these Black women would agree that because of their God talk, they are made stronger, as Black women and as Black women surviving breast cancer.

TRANSFORMING CONVERSATIONS WITH GOD AND OTHERS—CANCER SURVIVORS' CHRISTIAN THEOLOGICAL TASKS AND REVELATION

For African American breast cancer survivors who identify as Christian, theology is evidenced as faith that seeks and asks questions of a living God. This living God is simultaneously a transcendent God who is revealed, yet ever remains a mystery at times beyond their human understanding.[12] These survivors' inquiries about God come from, first, an ontological awareness of God as the creator and redeemer of all things. This God, which as theists they view as approachable, loving, and present, reveals God-self through scripture. Their inquiries also emanate out of faith in God, not, as Migliore points out, in an "attempt to arrive at certainty apart from God."[13] No, Black breast cancer survivors' awareness of God does not happen apart from talking to and living life with God. Therefore, Christian theology as part of the cultural logic of African American Christian faith is conversational.[14] It happens in conversations with others and God. Thus as one African American breast cancer survivor described after being told her diagnosis over the phone, "The first thing I said when I hung up was, 'Lord, what did I do? But after that it was like, 'I need you. I need you to help me do this.' And that was my first conversation I would say after my diagnosis and after that we [God and I] had our 'conversations' is what I call it."

African American breast cancer survivors know God by talking to and living life with God. Conversation is the vehicle for questions to be raised. Conversations are also the means by which transformative work for African American cancer survivors happens.

For Black women dealing with breast cancer, there are many questions the disease raises for their Christian theology to grapple with. Some of these questions concern soteriology or salvation: “Where are you God?” “How will you save me from this?” Other questions center on mortality: “What happens after we die?” “Will I live to see my children grow up or accomplish the things I wanted to achieve in life?” Some focus on bodily integrity: “What has happened to my body?” “Am I a whole person now that I no longer have my breast(s)?” Others focus on theodicy and ask why breast cancer happened: “Was this punishment for something I did?” Still others seek meaning in the experience: “What does having breast cancer mean?” “Why did I experience breast cancer?” For some, the central theological questions breast cancer raises center on survivorship: “What does it mean now that I have survived breast cancer?” “Will life ever be normal again?” “What am I called to do having lived through cancer?”

At the core of these questions are concerns about “troubles” and God’s presence in the midst of troubles. These questions call for resources to answer them, as well as speak to Christian theology’s challenge to respond. Before considering the theological sources African American breast cancer survivors turn to for answers, let us first consider the Christian theological task Black breast cancer survivors undertake in seeking answers to their life questions and why they engage in the task of seeking answers.

Christian theology seeks to make meaning about God within the context of people’s lives, particularly their troubles. As Grenz and Erskine describes this meaning making, it calls for examining forms and symbols that cultural groups find meaningful.[15] Black breast cancer survivors’ narrative expressions are one set of forms and symbols they use to make meaning. Survivors’ words consequently provide the texts out of which their Christian theology is constructed. Black breast cancer survivors’ narratives reflect broader socially situated theologies that are not fixed but, as cultural processes, are developed through social interactions. African American breast cancer survivors actively orchestrate and are not just passive respondents to what happens to them.[16] Black breast cancer survivors’ constructive Christian theology happens in interactions/work with God, themselves, African American cancer survivors, and others. Consequently, Black breast cancer survivors do not just espouse their theology. They practice theology that is relevant to their lives and social circumstances.

A relevant theology that African American cancer survivors believe and practice is a culturally grounded one that articulates Christian beliefs in a language, manner, and thought forms understandable to people in the wider world to which Christianity ministers.[17] As an ethnographer and theologian, the job of articulating Black breast cancer survivors' practical and relevant theology occurs by translating what happens in African American cancer survivors' lives through the prism of Christian belief. What Black breast cancer survivors say about resolving problems and articulate in their longings and desires reflects a broader cultural ethos of African American breast cancer survivors.

At the core of Black breast cancer survivors' theology is affirmation of hope in God. Their hope is in a transcendent God who is forever loving, redeeming, and transformative in the midst of breast cancer's troubles and all the troubles they face. This God is the one borne out of the tradition of Christian Black women, in the past, for whom Jesus was their central frame of reference. These Black women identified with Jesus out of his humanity, because they believed Jesus identified with them. As Jesus suffered undeservedly, so Black women suffered cruelty. This Jesus, whose suffering culminated in crucifixion, is the one Black women, under chattel slavery, identified with through their experiences of rape and sexual violation, economic exploitation, in seeing their families destroyed and children sold away, and who survived despite their freedom being denied to them. This Jesus, as part of the trinity, understood as God or the divine incarnate, was the one Black women believed would respond to their struggles and pains.[18] This is the God contemporary Black women, as part of a womanist theological tradition, inherited from their foremothers through chattel slavery, post-slavery and reconstruction, segregation and Jim Crow, the civil rights movement, and into the twentieth and twenty-first centuries. This womanist faith of their foremothers is part of the secure base and safe haven (along with God) Black women attach their hope in God to. Because Black women throughout history have trusted in God and prevailed against the odds, contemporary Black women with breast cancer can be assured and confident that they, too, can trust in God.[19]

Katie Ernst calls the hope these Black breast cancer survivors demonstrate "complex hope."[20] Complex hope is the act of naming the intense and often terrifying reality of the present while also demanding the possibility of a different future from one's surrounding community. The act of hoping, from this definition, transforms the reality of the present.[21] Black women in this study deal with the present and terrifying reality that they will die from breast cancer. Yet, they envision a different future for themselves, a future without breast cancer. Because surviving breast cancer is a possibility, Black women use this possibility to transform their reality. They act like breast cancer survivors because they see themselves as survivors.

This complex hope that Black women with breast cancer exhibit is different from what Ernst calls optimistic hope, which is goal-setting hope, centered in individualistic motivations to achieve desired goals and ends through individual progression and trust in one's abilities.[22] Black women with breast cancer, while able to act on their own, believe that what it takes to survive breast cancer is more than they can provide for themselves alone. Their complex hope is also different from eschatological or future-oriented hope, which is an escapist hope that avoids present reality in hopes of something better in the next life.[23] While Black women do envision being healed of breast cancer after death (and often talk about those who die from breast cancer as finally healed at the point of their deaths), the Black women in this study are not satisfied with freedom from breast cancer in the hereafter or time to come. No, they seek healing from breast cancer in the present and struggle in the present with God to attain it. Attuned to their reality, Black women turn to God and their faith to center their hope.

Hope, of the type these Black women with breast cancer have, as the womanist theologian A. Elaine Brown Crawford further explains is "the theological construct that moves women beyond endurance to survival, and ultimately, toward the transformation of oppressive circumstances. Hope is the bridge from oppression to liberation that facilitates fully humanity and fosters an undaunted passion for life."[24]

This act of hope for Crawford is defined through the "holler," or the refusal of Black women to remain silent to the suffering they experience. The holler, which can be exhibited through Black women's public sharing of suffering with others, breast cancer testimonies, public advocacy for Black women to be screened for breast cancer, and Black women's literal crying out, is a holler that demands recognition to be seen, heard, and attended to. The act of hollering, which gives rise to these Black women's complex hope, requires that Black women with breast cancer take risks and expose themselves to vulnerability to voice their suffering.[25] Their hope develops out of a process instigated by stress and suffering.[26] Breast cancer as a life-threatening menace that generates both stress and suffering for Black women who experience it, particularly until Black women use their faith to confront both. Complex hope, as Ernst says, "is a matter of life or death for the individual [Black woman with breast cancer] to thrive, versus merely survive."[27]

African American breast cancer survivors' hope in God is therefore hope that deals with their real challenges, struggles, desires, and questions. Answers to their fundamental theological questions come from many texts—namely, scripture and experience. African American cancer survivors interpret these texts out of their cultural experiences as Black woman, the Black Church religious experience, and African American biblical hermeneutics. Grant identifies the Bible to be a major resource for the religious validation of Black women's lives. God's revelation as witnessed through the Bible, which Black women historically (and contemporarily) read and hear in the context of their experiences, along with God's revelation directly to them, serve as key components of Black women's God-consciousness and are reflective of a womanist theological tradition.[28]

Scripture, as Migliore describes, "is the unique and irreplaceable witness to the liberating and reconciling activity of God in the history of Israel and supremely in Jesus Christ. By the power of the Holy Spirit, Scripture serves the purpose of relating [people] to God and transforming [their] lives."[29] Scripture bears witness for Black breast cancer survivors to an ever-present God in the midst of changing temporal, corporate, and personal circumstances. For these cancer survivors, troubles come, but God remains the same. Scripture confirms this. This is the reason why Bernice,[30] an African American breast cancer survivor in conversation with other Black breast cancer survivors, says,

> I may sound strange. I want to know, "What does the Bible say about it?" I want to go from that angle. I want to believe and trust that it will be better even those days when I don't feel. My feelings can't always dictate everything. Feelings come and go. They change like the weather, [others agree in the background] swinging here and there. What can I stand on that's solid? [She pounds on the table.] That regardless to this, regardless God will yet exist. Life will yet be. It is going to get better. I want to hold onto something. Am I making sense? Is what I'm saying making sense?

Indeed what Bernice is asking for makes sense. She turns to the Bible because for her it functions as a witness of God's stable and immutable presence.

For African American breast cancer survivors, Biblical witness, which is located in scripture, points to an ever-present and caring God, a God whose grace does not forsake them in their times of need.[31] As Bernice's statements reflect, as a Christian, she does not just "believe *in* the Bible" to change her situation; she "believes in the living God attested *by* the Bible" to change her situation by giving her right perspective.[32] As Migliore asserts that, seen in this way, "Scripture is indispensable in bringing [people] into a new relationship with the living God through Christ by the power of the Holy Spirit, and thus into new relationship with others and the entire creation."[33] God's presence and ontological nature are revealed for Black breast cancer survivors through scripture. These revelations of God are not static, but understood through their lived experiences of God as part of a womanist theological tradition. As a consequence, for African American breast cancer survivors, experience is a particularly vital cultural resource for articulating their Christian theology.

Lived experience provides material to understand scripture. In line with Peters's criterion for systematic theology,[34] whether or not one's theological position holds up against the collective body of knowledge people have accumulated through living is an important measurement by which to judge the validity of what is known about God.[35] Experience, or what Jones calls "lived, imaginative constructs," is what shapes the ways African American breast cancer survivors see themselves, those they are in relationship with, as well as understand their faith.[36] Black breast cancer survivors' experiences are influenced by culture. Black women's cultural foremothers relied on faith in God understood through lived experience, which created a tradition of womanist theology Black women with breast cancer continue to rely upon to draw meaning from scripture.

Therefore when Bernice shared her desire to know, "What does the Bible say about it?" her statements resonated with other African American breast cancer survivors she was in conversation with. These other survivors responded to what was said based on their shared cultural experiences as Black women, the Black Church tradition they are a part of, and womanist tradition of reading scripture in relation to lived experience they are heirs to. These shared cultural experiences, tradition, and reading of scripture form a collective African American biblical hermeneutic. This shared, interpretive framework gives these survivors similar assurances of God's faithfulness in their lives. The "terrain" of their lives, layered histories, and experiences as women of color, touched in similar and different ways by breast cancer, simultaneously converged in Bernice's testimony and the other survivors' responses to her statement. The convergence of their lived experiences, histories and cultures created a "localized thick description" and a particular understanding of scripture, experience, and culture as ways God reveals God's self to Black breast cancer survivors.[37]

As Erskine rightly notes, scripture, experience, and culture are not "different moments of the Spirit's speaking and hence [people's] listening. Rather, just as the Spirit who speaks is one Spirit, also the Spirit's speaking is one speaking."[38] The other Black breast cancer survivors in this exchange heard what Bernice said through filters of their own experiences and readings of scripture. Nevertheless, they also believed it was the same Holy Spirit speaking to all of them through her witness of God's power and authority in scripture. It was the transcendent power of the Holy Spirit, they believed, that changed her perspective about life, giving her access to new truths through biblical scripture. God's power for these Black breast cancer survivors continually converged in meaningful ways to help them know ontologically about God—who God is and how God works.

GOD AS TRANSFORMING LOVE: THE ECONOMIC AND IMMANENT TRINITY FOR BREAST CANCER

Ontological questions about God, namely *who God is* and *how God works*—are not easy questions for Black breast cancer survivors who identify with a womanist theological tradition to fully answer. God, although revealed to them, nevertheless remains a mystery. Yet, at the core of God, they believe, is "love," which has the power to transform their lives. As Migliore describes, "The God known in Jesus Christ by the Holy Spirit is God over [people], God for [people] and God in [people]—the loving God, the gracious Lord Jesus Christ, and the communion-creating spirit of God."[39] This triune God, the one Black women understand through scripture, reason, tradition, and experience, is one that African American breast cancer survivors, as heirs to a womanist theological tradition and nurtured in Black Church communities of faith, have constructed over time.[40] Although a cultural construction, the doctrine of the Trinity is important for womanist theology, particularly one relevant for African American women affected by breast cancer.

In the face of breast cancer, which causes early death for many Black women, a God who affirms life is important. Belief in a God who affirms life is central to a theology of well-being for these survivors. Although believing in a creative and sovereign God to many Black breast cancer survivors is comforting, it does not completely satisfy. For African American breast cancer survivors, a God who is merely sovereign can too easily be detached from their daily lives. For these survivors, a God who is sovereign yet who, as God made flesh, suffers and struggles with them, advocates for and is working in them, is more expansive and life renewing.[41] For them, this is a God who conquers death by giving life.[42] A God who can be all these things is a safe haven in times of trouble, reassuring African American breast cancer survivors that they are never alone. It also affirms for these cancer survivors that God is a transcendent being who is not static, but active. God, as a sovereign, advocating being who works within them, is a God who lives, moves, and transforms their human challenges, including cancer. The doctrine of the Trinity, as Migliore describes captures all these attributes of God. As he states,

> The doctrine of the Trinity redescribes God in the light of the event of Jesus Christ and the outpouring of God's transforming Spirit. It wants to say that God is sovereign, costly love liberates and renews life. It wants to say that God's love for the world in Christ now at work by the power of the Spirit is not accidental or capricious or temporary. It wants to say that there is no sinister or even demonic side of God . . . God is self-expending, other-affirming, community-building love.[43]

The doctrine of the Trinity as articulated by Black breast cancer survivors reflects that God's presence as three-in-one is an intimate presence. It also evidences to them that God is a being who is relational, to God's self and with them. God is in community with Black women with breast cancer. These aspects of the Trinity are important for African American breast cancer survivors in their reliance on God as a secure base and safe haven and in making meaning of what "having cancer" is about.

Talking about the triune God, Marlo, an African American breast cancer survivor, characterizes God as a three-in-one "being."[44] As she describes, "There's a God that's in me, the Holy Spirit that he said, 'Okay you have this. But you take a negative and make it positive.' And the Lord said, 'It's not your story. You share it. I'm going to let you be a light so you can share it.'" Marlo's doctrine of the Trinity is clear when she references God as "God, Holy Spirit, and Lord." Not separate beings, Marlo views God as three-in-one and as a community with whom she interacts and in which she plays a role. Being in community with God is important to Black breast cancer survivors, especially for those trying to maintain the Strong Black woman persona. For these in particular there are few with whom they can unburden, therefore God as their sole secure base truly function as "all in all."

The ways Marlo describes the triune God working in her life are suggestive of how Migliore describes God as "self-expending, other-affirming, community-building love."[45] Viewed through the lens of the Trinity, breast cancer is not something Marlo wanted. Nevertheless, breast cancer is something purposeful, life affirming, and community building because of what the triune God has/can/is doing through her. Marlo identifies the Godhead as a three-in-one community. In the same way Migliore speaks of the triune God as loving, Marlo speaks of God as transformative love, one who turns negatives into positives. God as transformative love, which is similar to how Migliore and Marlo describe God, further evidences clearly God as both an immanent and economic Trinity.

An immanent God refers to the ontological being of God. The immanent Trinity is the Godhead outside of time and space.[46] This is the God who speaks in Genesis 1 saying, "Let there be." Augustine's description of the Trinity is similar to Marlo's immanent and boundless conceptualization of God. The Trinity, for Augustine, is one who functions as "mutually related persons, existing in unity of equal essence."[47] Augustine means by this that the immanent Trinity functions not as an idea, but as a perpetually active force. For Marlo, and for many Black women with breast cancer drawing from a womanist theological tradition, the triune God is an ever-active force. Augustine uses the analogy of "lover," "beloved," and "love" to convey God's boundlessness as simultaneously the subject, object, and medium of God's love. Marlo does something similar when she speaks of herself as being the recipient of God's Holy Spirit, the agent of the spirit (i.e., through her testimony), and the embodied spirit (i.e., the light). For Marlo, only a transformative God could allow her to be all three at the same time.

Augustine's description of the immanent Trinity, similar to Marlo's articulation of God's power in/through her, is also what Cone, drawing from the

Black liberation theology tradition (of which womanist theology is an heir), says about God in Christ, as a member of the Trinity. As he notes, "Jesus Christ is not a proposition, not a theological concept that exists merely in our heads. He is an event of liberation, a happening in the lives of oppressed people."[48] God is transformative love, which liberates the oppressed. Black breast cancer survivors constitute those who are "oppressed" by "dynamic forces, both personal and social, that diminish or deny their flourishing."[49] Breast cancer is only one force that oppresses them. African American breast cancer survivors are also challenged by the intersectional oppressions of racism, sexism, and classism that affect every aspect of their lives, including their breast cancer diagnosis, treatment, and survivorship.

Breast cancer and the treatments these African American cancer survivors regularly endure often make them sick to the point of giving up. The disease and treatment, at times, denies their flourishing. Yet, these African American cancer survivors believe in an immanent Trinity, one who happens in the midst of their sickness. The Trinity is the liberating moments in the midst of cancer's troubles. As one survivor, Cheryl, describes going through chemotherapy,

> I literally could have died. It was a choice that I made. I chose to live in Christ versus, you know, stop eating, stop drinking, all the things. But I made a choice because I'm like, "Okay God. I know you've got something else for me." But then again that scripture came to mind, "I can do all things through Christ who strengthens me."[50]

Although Cheryl could have given up, she says she "chose to live in Christ." She chose to believe in the liberating activity of God to intervene in her situation. Her complex hope was in Christ to help her. Recalling the words of the apostle Paul, words from another historical period and cultural context, she speaks these life-affirming words into her present situation. As Meeks describes, Cheryl's cultural interpretation of this scripture is literal.[51] She took the scripture at face value and applied it to her circumstance. Her doing both is theologically sound. The way Cheryl speaks of "choosing to live in Christ" is similar to Cone's description of God's immanence as liberating love not bound by a particular place or time. God's love, as Cone theorizes out of a Black liberation theology and Cheryl articulates as heir to a womanist theological tradition, is a transcendent and transformational force.

God as "immanent Trinity" is closely related to what scholars also term God as being. That is God as an "economic Trinity."[52] Instead of just an ontological awareness of God, an economic Trinity is a way of characterizing God according to how God orders affairs and how this order is made known in history and human experience.[53] For Black breast cancer survivors, God as "economic Trinity" is practical and experienced in daily living. The Trinity as three-in-one is made evident in the story of the Israelites in Exodus. In this historical situation, God appears as liberator, the one who comes to the weak and oppressed, identifying with them, and transforming their enslaved existence into a liberated one.[54] The Israelites experience setbacks, yet God ultimately delivers them to their promised land. This is an idea similarly shared by some African American breast cancer survivors.

Anita, a sixty-something-year-old African American cancer survivor who underwent a mastectomy, chemotherapy, and reconstruction surgery following her diagnosis, uses the experience of the Israelites and God's ordering of affairs to interpret her own experience as a cancer survivor.[55]

> My motto is, "A setback is a setup for a comeback." And that's the way I have always looked at this condition. Spiritually, I sought out or people sought me out to give me this book . . . [that] talked about the situation of the Israelites who wandered to get to Canaan. And the fact that they had to wander for forty years, rather than forty days . . . because of their inability to accept God's decision and direction for their lives and the path [God] wanted them to go in, [God] allowed them to wander for so long. So I read that book and I got a better understanding of what this diagnosis meant to me and understood that sometimes we are used as channels for other people.

For Anita, God as an economic Trinity, uses her breast cancer experience for a purpose, a channel to reach other people. It serves as a means to help her talk to others, including those in her family, about their struggles with health challenges, including cancer and depression. For Anita, God's economy is one that takes "setbacks" like her diagnosis with breast cancer and transforms them into "setups for comebacks." Although for Anita the triune God is at work, she, like many other African American breast cancer survivors, also particularly draw strength from identifying with Jesus, as savior and friend, and from the Holy Spirit, which empowers her to listen and encourage others. Jesus and the Holy Spirit, as part of a transcendent and present God, become additional resources for making meaning of the breast cancer experiences.

JESUS A LIBERATING FRIEND—TRANSFORMING YESTERDAY, TODAY, AND WHAT IS TO COME

If breast cancer were the only challenge African American breast cancer survivors had to deal with, then that would be more than enough. Yet, it is not. These Black cancer survivors deal with a myriad of troubles. Some of these include abandonment by friends and loved ones after their diagnoses, fears about recurrence, stigma, and marginalization from employers who view requests for reasonable work accommodations as nuisances, pain management issues, fatigue, financial challenges, insurance disruptions, sadness about what their bodies look like following surgeries, hair loss, insomnia, cognitive disruptions, lymphedema, and cultural erasure within mainstream breast cancer survivor organizations that often fail to reflect their experiences—namely, as women of color touched by breast cancer.

All of these are just some of the breast cancer troubles these African American cancer survivors face. Many of these troubles are further complicated by racism, sexism, and economic elitism that not only affect them at work and home, but also in cancer survivorship. For a relevant and practical theology to meet these African American breast cancer survivors' needs, it has to be one that can "hear" and "identify with" their troubles and pain. To invigorate a hope that believes in the power of God to transform oppressive situations, hope for African American breast cancer survivors has to evidence a God that understands the troubles these women go through. As previously mentioned, a God that simply watches over is not sufficient for a sustained hope in the troubles African American breast cancer survivors face. Only a God that can function "over," "for," and "in" these African American cancer survivors' troubles will suffice. It is through the incarnate Christ that God "for" Black women with breast cancer becomes particularly evident.

Because the imminence and economy of the triune God is love not limited by time or space, yet tangible enough to meet present needs, it requires a Christology that is past, present, and future oriented. Jesus Christ for these Black breast cancer survivors is the embodiment of God's boundless love. Cone aptly characterizes this Christology as, "Jesus is who he was," "Jesus is who he is,"[56] and "Jesus is who he will be."[57] For these breast cancer survivors, Jesus who lived, died and rose again is significant because he is the one who can identify with their struggles. Not out of his maleness, but his humanity, Jesus is the one who healed others who were sick. As Cheryl, a forty-year-old breast cancer survivor who underwent a lumpectomy and radiation shared during an exchange with other survivors,[58]

> I think personally for me there is a scripture in Philippians 4, "I can do all things through Christ who strengthens me." And then there is another scripture in the Bible talking about the woman with the issue of blood for twelve years. [Others agree in the background.] And I thought about it. I mean we all have issues. We all have something. In this particular case now it's cancer. But we all have some issue.

For Cheryl identifying with this Jesus and what he can do starts by identifying with what Jesus has done. Understanding Jesus is linked to history and who Jesus was.

Jesus, as a soteriological figure or one who saves, is located in the history of the Israelites who Yahweh covenants with, and who is the fulfillment of Jewish messianic prophecies.[59] As recorded in Luke 4:18–19, Jesus is anointed by God and empowered by the Holy Spirit to bring good news to the poor, proclaim release for captives, restore sight to the blind, release those in bondage, and proclaim the entrance of God's favor.[60] The Synoptic gospels and John, just as Cheryl recalls in the biblical passage of the hemorrhagic woman described in Mark 5:21–34 and Luke 8:40–48, provide witness to Jesus's performance of these works. Jesus's acts identify him as a liberator. For Cheryl, Jesus's liberation is notably identified with healing.

Jesus's presence as liberator in the gospels affirms for her Jesus's humanity and connects Jesus's story with God's liberation of the Israelites from slavery in Egypt as recorded in Exodus.[61] Jesus represents for Cheryl the constancy of God's liberating power. Just as God liberated the Israelites from bondage in Egypt, God, through Jesus, came yet again to liberate humanity. The incarnate Christ is the basis on which Cheryl and other Black cancer survivors can believe in the redemptive power of the triune God to save the world from evil, sin, and death. Jesus's incarnation is the secure base, safe haven, and bridge that connect them to God.[62] Yet, Jesus is more than just human to these African American breast cancer survivors. Jesus is also divine.

As divine, Jesus is also for them the "beloved" of God.[63] Anointed as "Christ" or "Messiah" sent by God, Jesus embodies the triune God's economy, which is transformative love for the world.[64] Therefore, as Cone argues, Jesus, as part of the Black liberation theological tradition (and womanist theological tradition) is more than a historical figure. Jesus, as God's love incarnate, is a recurring event, just as God's liberation is.[65] In the present, Jesus is the crucified Christ, the divine one who steps into Black people's human situations. The cross, as part of Jesus's story, Meeks identifies as being what makes Jesus the "center of Christian faith."[66] This is what Cheryl and the other African American breast cancer survivors believe in. They believe in the crucified Christ. The cross, in turn, becomes for them the tangible symbol of Jesus's suffering.

It is through the cross that the triune God, through Jesus Christ, identifies with human suffering.[67] Jesus's service as Christ crucified and the risen Lord are what locate the triune God in the present. Therefore, when Cheryl speaks of "Christ who strengthens me," she is not talking merely about the historical Jesus who healed the bleeding woman in the scriptures. Nor is she speaking only about the Christ who died and was buried. She is talking about Jesus Christ in the present tense, the one who rose and appeared to Mary Magdalene.[68] The resurrected Jesus gives her and other African American breast cancer survivors fortitude as their safe haven to deal with cancer and other challenges they encounter. If Jesus overcame suffering, death and the grave, Cheryl believes as an African American woman she can endure breast cancer with "Christ's strength" and all that comes with it. This ability to keep going for these cancer survivors is also eschatologically connected to Jesus as the one "who will be."

This Jesus "who will be" is the one coming again in the future to finally resolve the struggle over suffering, death, and the challenges Cheryl and other African American breast cancer survivors experience in the present.[69] This is the "Coming Lord" as Cone terms him.[70] This eschatological view embedded in Black liberation and womanist theologies envisions Jesus as coming again to establish the reign of the triune God for good. For those who are suffering with illness and oppression, this coming Jesus represents a final conquering of death and disease; Jesus is the awakening of a new age.

For these Black breast cancer survivors, this coming Christ is the "eschatological moment" envisioned as their and other "women's wholeness" and "a bold vision of what life without oppression might be like."[71] More than eschatological or escapist hope, this belief in what is yet to come, as part of complex hope, also gives these survivors the courage to continuing surviving. They truly believe God is not through with them yet. This faith in what is yet to be for them is essential to their ideas about well-being. Therefore, as Marlo, a breast cancer survivor diagnosed with late stage breast cancer in her forties, told a gathering of cancer survivors,

> Taken everything that I have lived through even when I just could have died, literally could have died, just died. But I said, "Okay Lord, I'm going to fight. . . . Just keep persevering. Just keep pushing. Just let the Lord lead me on this experience. And that's what I did. That's what helps get me through.

Marlo perseveres because she believes that something better is on the horizon for her. That hope in what is yet to come renews her when things are hard. She keeps pushing because she believes the Lord is with her in the struggle.

THE PRESENCE OF THE HOLY SPIRIT—TRANSFORMING POWER IN BREAST CANCER

In the face of statistics that indicate many African American breast cancer survivors will not live into old age and the personal challenges many of them face, what gives them the strength to continue? What gives Marlo the resolve to "fight back" against breast cancer? A simple answer would be the Holy Spirit, the additional member of the triune God. But to simply say that the Holy Spirit, as part of the triune God, does the work belies the fact that these survivors are active participants also in the work of the triune God in their lives. They believe the Holy Spirit does not just act upon them. They also believe it acts "in community" with them.

The Holy Spirit is for these African American breast cancer survivors an essential member of the intra-Trinitarian community.[72] In Black breast cancer survivors' lives, the Holy Spirit functions as a "rest on thing" person drawn into their material situations, who befriends their bodies, gives them strength to endure, and draws them (and all creation) into unity with the triune God. As Rogers points out, the Holy Spirit's ability to do this work of resting on, befriending, and drawing humanity is evident in the incarnate Christ.[73] It is why many of these Black cancer survivors mention Philippians 4:13 as a source of strength. It is the Holy Spirit operating through the incarnate Christ that strengthens them. The Holy Spirit at work makes Black cancer survivors' relationship with God as their secure base possible.

In the context of God's love, which is an ongoing and recurring event, the Holy Spirit functions in important ways in God's transformation of these survivors' lives. The Holy Spirit by "resting on" and befriending these Black women's bodies, liberates from what separates them from God (e.g., fear of death), transforms them into new beings, and allows them to assume a new way of living.[74] As Carlice Harris, another breast cancer survivor once told me, "When you are no longer afraid to die is when you truly start to live."[75] The Holy Spirit took away her fear of dying and the unknown. What it gave her in return was new insight and a new lease on life. Whatever time remains, she was going to live to the fullest.

As wisdom of God increases through African American breast cancer survivors' ongoing relationship with the triune God, the Holy Spirit continues its transformative work. The Holy Spirit, as Jesus promised in biblical scripture, is what guides these survivors into important truths about themselves in relationship with God.[76] Sandra, a fifty-five-year-old breast cancer survivor who underwent a mastectomy and reconstruction, affirms this when she shares,[77]

> I was with a friend for about three and a half years and he just dropped me cold turkey. . . . I think it made me stronger. And I think God has a way of doing things to make us realize that, "Hey, you are stronger than you think you are." And I think a lot of that really helped me to be a stronger person. [God] really made me stronger to kind of stand on my own and look to [God] for guidance and help.

These survivors' continued transformation or sanctification is the promise these Black women believe the Holy Spirit provides. This promise is that the redemptive work started by the triune God is guaranteed to continue until God's redemption of them is complete.[78]

African American cancer survivors, as others who identify with Jesus's death and resurrection, do so in the context of their cultural history in the United States and their current situations. This is what Cone says moves the Holy Spirit within Cheryl, making her call out to God saying, "Okay Lord.

I'm going to fight." It is also what moves Bernice to declare, "I do matter. I count. I am important. God put me in the world for a purpose." The Holy Spirit affirms their importance to the triune God. In God, these Black breast cancer survivors have an identity, a safe haven, and a home.[79] They know themselves as saved by God's grace, righteousness, and love.[80]

This acknowledgment of marginalized people's (e.g., African Americans') humanity and intrinsic worth is the cornerstone of a theology of complex hope in the Black religious experience.[81] It is the recognition that in the triune God, these women, even facing breast cancer, do matter to God. This Black cultural theology of complex hope says that what happened in the past, Jesus's overcoming of pain and death through the resurrection, is possible in the present in their struggles with breast cancer and will be finalized in the coming reign of God when their bodies are fully restored.[82]

When a theology of complex hope is connected to the person of Jesus, Cone contends it no longer functions as an intellectual idea. It becomes the praxis of freedom in oppressed communities.[83] As he says, "To hope in Jesus is to see the vision of his coming presence, and thus one is required by hope itself to live as if the vision is already realized in the present."[84] These breast cancer survivors in the midst of treatments reach out and encourage others. They support each other's well-being. Even when they are in pain, they organize galas to celebrate survivorship. Out of their pain, they act as change agents.[85] In community, these African American breast cancer survivors continually act as if they are already healed. They act as if they are whole because they believe an eschatology in which their bodies will be wholly resurrected.[86]

This same eschatological belief fueled by the Holy Spirit also gives these cancer survivors assurance that the triune God will see them through breast cancer. While they anticipate ultimate healing, they are simultaneously transformed by the breast cancer experience. They are forever changed and changing. As Roxanne, a breast cancer survivor in her late thirties who underwent a double mastectomy followed by reconstruction, says, "Yeah, I have been broken, but I have been put back together better than I ever was."[87] These African American breast cancer survivors see themselves being put back together as part of the triune God's ongoing work of redeeming creation. Yet, the work of being redeemed, these Black cancer survivors are aware, is not always easy. Breast cancer brings its share of hard days and troubles for these survivors also.

CREATED OUT OF NOTHING AND MADE IN THE IMAGE OF GOD—AN ESCHATOLOGICAL HOPE OF TRANSFORMATION IN BREAST CANCER

For African American breast cancer survivors, although God's creation is good, it is nevertheless imperfect.[88] Made in the image of the triune God (*imago Dei*), human beings are equally as imperfect and flawed. Yet it is *ex nihilo*—"out of nothing"—that God generated creation and all that is in it. The fact that the triune God created the world and its inhabitants out of God's self is key to African American breast cancer survivors' transformative theology of complex hope. God's creative power and its connection to a transformative theology of complex hope are important for three primary reasons—namely, God's act of creating out of nothing demonstrates for these cancer survivors God's love for creation. As Migliore points out, God's work of creation is "costly grace."[89] It is an act of divine *kenosis*. God's creative work empties out of self to make room for Black women's life.[90]

The doctrine of *ex nihilo* is also important because it underscores the world and Black women's dependence on God.[91] Because humans are made in the image of God, yet imperfect, suggests that the same God can (re)create humanity until all humanity fully reflects God. Thus this dependence on God suggests for African American breast cancer survivors a complex hope for creation's redemption. God will refashion creation until the final fulfillment of life is achieved. This hope in God's ongoing work of (re)creating creation is Black women's faith in grace that saves creation from sin, evil, and death.[92]

Lastly, the doctrine of creation "out of nothing" also evidences for African American breast cancer survivors an intimacy between God and creation. God's act of creation is not arbitrary, but purposeful.[93] God's creative work for Black women with breast cancer reflects a concurring providence between the triune God and creation.[94] God's covenant with creation is one in which God's providence provides what is needed and God's grace conforms to Black women's lives. God's grace activates the freedom of Black women with breast cancer, giving them new life.[95]

Each of these is important to a transformative theology of complex hope relevant to the experiences of African American breast cancer survivors. That God created life as a sacrificial act of love means that life and preserving life are important to God. Therefore anything contrary to what stands for life, Black women, as part of a womanist theological tradition, view as antithetical to God. Therefore, when these Black breast cancer survivors stand up for life by praying for others while actively taking chemotherapy, call each other to offer words of encouragement, or share their testimonies of being breast cancer survivors, they stand in solidarity with the creative work of God. African American breast cancer survivors in community with the triune

God and each other stand up for life and life's flourishing. In standing up for life they believe they are continually transformed to reflect the image of God.

The fact that these survivors credit their abilities to go through cancer treatment and surgeries, lose and regrow hair following chemotherapy, show people their mastectomy scars and reconstructed breasts, and reprioritize their lives by doing things that bring them joy bears witness to their total dependency on God and intimacy with God. God's grace through faith has conformed to these Black women survivors' lives in ways that has fit them for the cancer journey. As Constance, quoted at the beginning of the chapter says,

> I used to say, "Okay, Lord. You knew I could handle it. So. Okay. All right. This is what it is. And this is how we are going to deal with it." But I thank God it has been a journey. It has been an experience for sure. And I thank God for faith. [Others agree in the background.] Because if you don't have faith. A lot of times it is you and God having that conversation and nobody else.

These survivors' belief in a loving and covenantal God assures them that the triune God is on the cancer journey with them, empowering them to live and thrive beyond their cancer experiences. Being assured of God's presence is essential to dealing with the harsh realities of breast cancer and the ways it denies, limits, and seeks to wreak havoc in these survivors' lives.

Breast cancer and the troubles it brings are an evil force, namely because, as Meeks indicates, it does not have its own being, but instead, like evil, attaches parasitically, reducing its host to nothingness.[96] Breast cancer stands in opposition to what life stands for, which is the thriving of God's creation.[97] For those affected by breast cancer, recognizing breast cancer and its isolating effects as life destroying, is necessary for cultivating complex hope and struggling against physical, psychosocial, and spiritual death. These survivors know that breast cancer, if unchecked, can lead to their untimely physical deaths. Breast cancer uncontested can also lead to other forms of death, including psychic, spiritual, and emotional death. As Meeks describes, all of these types of death are fundamentally "the power of nothingness or that which makes empty and void."[98] For these Black breast cancer survivors, not standing up against breast cancer can easily lead to giving up on life. Death is something these breast cancer survivors actively struggle with.

These survivors are well acquainted with evil and the types of death breast cancer brings. This is particularly evident when they talk about their sadness and depression. As Renee, a seventy-something breast cancer survivor whose daughter died from breast cancer in her mid-thirties describes, "As everyone has pointed out, there is a time of sadness. Don't be fooled [others agree in the background] that you have not thought about death, have not thought about what this has done to your body and what it will mean for your relationships."[99] With these thoughts it is easy for survivors to give into sadness and allow breast cancer's evil and troubles to envelop them. This is what Eunice, a forty-five-year-old breast cancer survivor who underwent a mastectomy, calls "going behind the walls."[100] As she further describes,

> Behind those walls, it's nothing there. And if you are not thinking positive, reading something positive, you can get so depressed where you won't. You won't want to do to get dressed. You don't want to eat. You don't want to do nothing. And you can sleep all day, all night, a few days. So why go through that?

Not staying behind those "walls" requires African American cancer survivors to be reminded of God's grace that stands for them and God's covenant with them that calls them into community with God and others. These others with whom African American breast cancer survivors are in community even include those who have died from breast cancer.

Although Black breast cancer survivors affirm hope of bodily healing in the present, they are ever aware that death from breast cancer is a real possibility. Instead of naively denying death, they have found ways to incorporate death into the community of the living. One of the tangible ways this is done is by remembering, at public gatherings and events for African American breast cancer survivors, those who have died. Deceased cancer survivors' names are read aloud. The presence of these members is recalled in a way similar to how Mouw and Peters speak of ancestral presence as commemorated in some African cultures.[101] *Nommo*, or the generative power of the spoken word is also evident in these remembrance events in that calling the deceased person's name invokes their spirit to be present among the living.[102]

Although these remembrances evoke tears and sadness, they also inspire hope for these African American breast cancer survivors. They inspire complex hope because survivors who have died are not viewed as separated from the group, but instead part of the "great cloud of witnesses" Black breast cancer survivors believe are acknowledged in Hebrews 12:1. Deceased cancer survivors are seen by living cancer survivors as those restored to bodily wholeness and behind a veil that separates time from eternity, cheering on those still living to keep believing in God and striving for life. These deceased survivors become part of the hope-filled lineage of Black women that Black women who are still alive cling to.[103] Viewing deceased survivors in this way takes the sting out of death for African American cancer survivors.[104] These "living dead," as Mouw and Peters term them, give living African American cancer survivors examples of survivorship and faithfulness to pattern their own lives after. Even in other cancer survivors' deaths, Black breast cancer survivors' complex hope is renewed.

TRANSFORMED FOR GOD'S REDEEMING WORK OF HUMANITY: BREAST CANCER SURVIVORS AS ADVOCATES

For several African American breast cancer survivors who participated in this study, their advocacy was not something they chose for themselves. Instead it was something they were called to through their relationship with the triune God. Many see themselves as delivered from breast cancer in order to witness to others about God's redemptive grace. As Wanda, who underwent a lumpectomy shares, "I thought I have had a story to tell. But when I hear so many other stories everybody's story is unique . . . And we are here for a purpose. And that purpose is to keep going and to help the next person. So, I feel my experience will help someone else."[105] Renee[106] offered these additional thoughts,

> Each and every time I thought about that [things that made her depressed] I also thought about, "Oh this is my way to show that my God," that God that we all serve, is capable of bringing us back from the brink of depression, the brink of perhaps death and desperation within ourselves. And so we can reflect that to others whether it be in our speech, our mannerism, or ability to go and get involved in different activities that push us out front. I think that has helped me to recognize that my God . . . what you have done for me through this trial.

Wanda and Renee, like so many of their cancer survivor counterparts, believe they have been redeemed from breast cancer for a purpose. That purpose is to demonstrate God's love, grace, and power to overcome evil, sin, and death. Their God talk renews their strength by encouraging them to struggle against the troubles of breast cancer and to use their pain as the catalyst for their transformation. In survivorship they stand as "living witness" to the transformative and creative power of God to bring them back from the throes of breast cancer. These Black cancer survivors use their pain to generate and sustain their complex hope, a hope in God that does not turn away from breast cancer's pains and troubles, but motivates them as survivors to act, speak out (and holler if necessary) with assurance, "My God . . . what you have done for me through this trial."

NOTES

1. Constance is a pseudonym and all personal details of her life are fictionalized.
2. American Cancer Society. (2016). *Cancer Facts & Figures for African Americans 2016–2018.* Atlanta: American Cancer Society, 10.
3. Ibid., 4.
4. Ibid., 9.
5. Grant, J. (1989). *White Women's Christ and Black Women's Jesus: Feminist Christology and Womanist Response.* Atlanta: Scholars Press; and Cone, J. (2003). *God of the Oppressed.* Maryknoll, NY: Orbis Books.

6. Siegel, D., and Hartzell, M. (2003). *Parenting from the Inside Out: How a Deeper Self-Understanding Can Help You Raise Children Who Thrive.* New York: Penguin Group; and Crawford, A. E. (2002). *Hope in the Holler: A Womanist Theology.* Louisville, KY: Westminster John Knox Press.

7. Division of Christian Education of the National Council of Churches of Christ in the U.S.A. (1989). *New Revised Standard Version Bible.* New York: HarperCollins Publishers, Romans 8:28–30.

8. Jones, S. (2000). *Feminist Theory and Christian Theology: Cartographies of Grace.* Minneapolis: Augsburg Fortress.

9. Collins, P. H. (1998). *Fighting Words: Black Women and the Search for Justice.* Minneapolis: University of Minnesota Press.

10. Division of Christian Education. *New Revised Standard Version Bible*, Psalm 23.

11. Durkheim, E. (1976). *The Elementary Forms of the Religious Life.* (J. Wardwain, Trans.) London: George Allen & Unwin, 416.

12. Migliore, D. (2004). *Faith Seeking Understanding: An Introduction to Christian Theology.* Grands Rapids, MI: William B. Eerdmans, 3.

13. Ibid., 5.

14. Ibid.

15. Grenz, S. J., and Erskine, N. L. (2003). "How Do We Know What to Believe? Revelation and Authority." In W. C. Placher (Ed.), *Essentials of Christian Theology*, 20–32. Louisville, KY: Westminster John Knox Press.

16. Ibid., 31.

17. Ibid.

18. Grant. *White Women's Christ and Black Women's Jesus*, 212.

19. Ernst, K. (2017). "Terror of Hope: The Integration of Attachment Theory and Womanist Theology." *Pastoral Psychology*, *66*, 201–212.

20. Ibid., 202.

21. Ibid.

22. Ibid., 201; and Snyder, C. (2002). "Hope Theory: Rainbows in the Mind." *Psychological Inquiry*, *13* (4), 249–275.

23. Ernst. "Terror of Hope," 202; and Moltmann, J. (1967). *Theology of Hope: On the Ground and the Implications of Christian Eschatology.* Minneapolis: Fortress Press.

24. Crawford. *Hope in the Holler*, xii.

25. Ibid.

26. Ernst. "Terror of Hope," 207.

27. Ibid., 203.

28. Grant. *White Women's Christ and Black Women's Jesus*, 211.

29. Migliore. *Faith Seeking Understanding*, 44.

30. Bernice is a pseudonym and all personal details of her life are fictionalized.

31. Meeks, Douglas. (2012). "The Authority and Criticism of Scripture." Lecture presented DIV 2656, Constructive Christian Theology, Nashville, September 2012.

32. Migliore. *Faith Seeking Understanding*, 50.

33. Ibid.

34. Peters, Ted. (2015). *God—The World's Future: Systematic Theology for the New Era.* 3rd ed. Minneapolis: Augsburg Fortress.

35. Meeks, Douglas. (2012). "Knowing God: Sources and Norms: Scripture, Tradition, Reason and Experience." Lecture presented DIV 2656, Constructive Christian Theology, Nashville, September 2012.

36. Jones. *Feminist Theory and Christian Theology.*

37. Ibid., 37–39.

38. Grenz and Erskine. "How Do We Know What to Believe?," 33.

39. 69.

40. Ibid., 67.

41. Division of Christian Education. *New Revised Standard Version Bible*, John 3:31–36.

42. Ibid., Romans 8:9–11.

43. Migliore. *Faith Seeking Understanding*, 72.

44. Marlo is a pseudonym and all personal details of her life are fictionalized.
45. Migliore. *Faith Seeking Understanding*, 72.
46. McGrath, Alister. (2007). "The Doctrine of the Trinity." In *Christian Theology: An Introduction*, 4th ed. Oxford: Blackwell, 253.
47. Augustine. (2011). "On the Trinity." In Alister McGrath (Ed.), *The Christian Theology Reader*. Malden, MA: Wiley-Blackwell, 165.
48. Cone, James. (2003). *God of the Oppressed*. Maryknoll, NY: Orbis, 32.
49. Jones. *Feminist Theory and Christian Theology*, 71.
50. Cheryl is quoting Philippians 4:13 (Division of Christian Education. *New Revised Standard Version Bible*, Philippians 4:13).
51. Meeks. "The Authority and Criticism of Scripture."
52. McGrath. "The Doctrine of the Trinity," 253.
53. Ibid.
54. Marbury, H. (2015). *Pillars of Cloud and Fire: The Politics of Exodus in African American Biblical Interpretation.* New York: New York University Press; and Cone. *God of the Oppressed*, 71.
55. Anita is a pseudonym and all personal details of her life are fictionalized.
56. Cone. *God of the Oppressed*, 106, 110.
57. Ibid.,109.
58. Cheryl is a pseudonym and all personal details of her life are fictionalized.
59. Cone. *God of the Oppressed*, 109.
60. Migliore. *Faith Seeking Understanding*, 175.
61. Cone. *God of the Oppressed*, 109.
62. Ibid., 110.
63. Augustine. "On the Trinity."
64. Division of Christian Education. *New Revised Standard Version Bible*, John 3:16–21.
65. Cone. *God of the Oppressed*, 32.
66. Meeks, Douglas. (2012). "Jesus Christ—Questions." Lecture presented DIV 2656, Constructive Christian Theology, Nashville, October 16, 2012.
67. Ibid.
68. Division of Christian Education. *New Revised Standard Version Bible*, John 20:11–18.
69. Cone. *God of the Oppressed*, 116.
70. Ibid., 119.
71. Jones. *Feminist Theory and Christian Theology*, 75.
72. Rogers, Eugene. (2005). "Where the Spirit Rests: Matter and Narrative," In *After the Spirit: A Constructive Pneumatology from Resources Outside the Western World.* Grand Rapids, MI: William B. Eerdmans Publishing, 58.
73. Ibid., 60–61.
74. Migliore. *Faith Seeking Understanding*, 228.
75. Carlice Harris is a pseudonym and all personal details of her life are fictionalized.
76. Division of Christian Education. *New Revised Standard Version Bible*, John 16:12–15.
77. Sandra is a pseudonym and all personal details of her life are fictionalized.
78. Migliore. *Faith Seeking Understanding*, 229.
79. Meeks, Douglas. (2012). "Redemption." Lecture presented DIV 2656, Constructive Christian Theology, Nashville, November 8, 2012.
80. Ibid.
81. Ibid., 117.
82. Ibid.
83. Ibid., 118.
84. Migliore. *Faith Seeking Understanding*, 119.
85. Townes, E. (1993). "Living in the New Jerusalem: The Rhetoric and Movement of Liberation in the House of Evil." In *A Troubling in My Soul: Womanist Perspectives on Evil & Suffering*, 78–91. Maryknoll, NY: Orbis Books.
86. Division of Christian Education. *New Revised Standard Version Bible*, 1 Corinthians 15:35– 58.
87. Roxanne is a pseudonym and all personal details of her life are fictionalized.

88. Migliore. Faith Seeking Understanding, 103.
89. Ibid., 101.
90. Ibid.
91. Ibid.
92. Ibid., 102.
93. Ibid., 105.
94. Meeks, Douglas. (2012). "Creation." Lecture presented DIV 2656, Constructive Christian Theology, Nashville, November 1, 2012.
95. Ibid.
96. Ibid.
97. Ibid.
98. Ibid.
99. Renee is a pseudonym and all personal details of her life are fictionalized.
100. Eunice is a pseudonym and all personal details of her life are fictionalized.
101. Mouw, R. J., and Peters, T. (2003). "Where are we going? Eschatology." In W. C. Placher (Ed.), *Essentials of Christian Theology*. Louisville: Westminster John Knox Press, 350.
102. Jackson, R., and Richardson, E. (Eds.). (2003). *Understanding African American Rhetoric: Classical and Contemporary Innovations.* New York: Routledge.
103. Ernst. "Terror of Hope," 204.
104. Division of Christian Education. *New Revised Standard Version Bible*, 1 Corinthians 15:54–56.
105. Wanda is a pseudonym and all personal details of her life are fictionalized.
106. Renee is a pseudonym and all personal details of her life are fictionalized.

Conclusion

Christian theology at its core is a story about how an active God intervenes in the lives of those who are in trouble, saving them from the troubles they face. What the troubles are being faced, who faces these troubles, where and how God intervenes, and how those who believe in God respond to God's intervention are the interests of both theology and anthropology. Theology seeks to know who God is and how God operates. Anthropology wants to know for what intents and purposes does God operate and what does God's operating mean for those who believe in God. This theological study, informed by anthropology, has sought to do both. Drawing from the Christian theological tradition evidenced in womanist theology, this study has focused its attention on the theology of African American women with breast cancer who see, know, pray to, talk to, struggle with, and understand God out of their experiences as Black women affected by race, class, and gender oppression.[1]

Because Black women with breast cancer experience race, class, and gender oppression, this study draws from anthropology in considering how these oppressions affect Black women and their experience of breast cancer. This is in keeping with what anthropology as a discipline does—namely, to study human beings in their totality, unrestricted by dimensions of space and time, with an emphasis on understanding the impact of social inequalities and reflecting cultural relativism in scholarship that it produces.[2] For anthropologists, understanding how social inequalities affect human beings and the cultural products they generate—namely, the theology Black women with breast cancer produce—requires reading across literature from diverse fields. This study has employed research from public health/biomedicine, feminist theory, leadership studies, African American women's history, and theology to understand the theology of Black women with breast cancer. What it also requires, which is a hallmark of the anthropology, is engaging in ethnographic research.

Ethnographic research, which includes collecting primary data from those whose life ways are of interest, is what grounds the connections and inferences that I as a theologian and anthropologist have made between what Black women with breast cancer think about God, say about God, and consequently do based on their faith in God. This study has benefited from conducting ethnographic interviews and focus groups and engaging in participant observation as a professional anthropologist, theologian, and pastor for more than fifteen years in varied social contexts, including Black breast cancer survivors support groups, churches, and homes. Listening to what Black women say about God and what their theology means to their lives are important areas for anthropological and theological inquiry.

Where the emphases of both womanist Christian theology and womanist anthropology as practiced here dovetail is in the primacy given to Black women's lives, experiences, challenges and thoughts. Womanist anthropology, in common with womanist theology, is committed to the intentional effort to bring the experiences of African American women center stage in scholarly research.[3] By directly considering how race, class, and gender oppression shape Black women's experiences and what those women do as social actors in responding to breast cancer, such work makes clear the richness of Black women's lives and cultural expressions. Even Black women's theology reflects this richness. What these streams have led to is a study of the theology of Black women and breast cancer reflected in these pages. This theology is grounded in a complex hope, a hope, which Black women inherited from their foremothers, that faces trouble, believes in God, and uses pain as the sustenance for leadership and survival.

African American women facing breast cancer face a disease that is a menace. It is a menace that brings trouble, from the very lethal nature of certain breast cancer types to aggressiveness among certain women, especially younger Black women. When breast cancer comes to Black women, it brings troubles by blocking access to screening, inhibiting access to quality care and treatment, preventing access to adequate insurance coverage to pay for care, and determining where and from whom Black women receive their breast cancer care. Breast cancer also brings troubles because of what it does to Black women's bodies and their relationships. The disease results in Black women's bodies being cut, disfigured, and scarred. Breast cancer disrupts Black women's relationships with their families and friends, with themselves and their bodies, and even with God. Breast cancer spells trouble for far too many Black women.

If breast cancer were the only trouble Black women faced, then it might in some ways not be so bad. But it is not. Breast cancer gets intertwined with other troubles Black women face as a consequence of being Black, female, and socioeconomically challenged. The intersectionality of Black women's lives ones is one in which African Americans face the intersecting troubles racism, sexism, and class oppression also bring.[4] These troubles make it more likely that African American women will be at increased risk for breast cancer because of the toxic environments in which they live. Intersectional oppressions make it more likely that Black women will literally carry the weight of their troubles on their bodies, leading to their greater risk for obesity and other comorbidities, which set them up for higher rates of breast cancer mortality. The trouble of being Black and female in a world that does not value either of them will mean that Black women will more likely be treated by health-care providers who neither respect them nor view them as responsible agents capable of following medical protocols to treat their breast cancers or sustain their lives. These, too, are the troubles that Black women with breast cancer confront.

Yet, trouble can't last always. Troubles necessitate a response. For many Black women that response is found in their faith and their womanist Christian theology. Their faith in God, which is grounded in their womanist Christian theology, is Black women's response to breast cancer. Their womanist Christian theology responds to trouble by declaring that the triune God (God, Jesus Christ, and the Holy Spirit) is a divine and active force that shows up to face trouble. This triune God faces Black women's troubles head on, promising to walk with Black women through the wilderness of breast cancer's troubles. This is a definitively womanist Christian theology cultivated in the Black churches and faith traditions many Black women grew up with and still participate in. This womanist Christian theology, while critical of sexism evident in the Black church tradition and of racism in white feminist theologies,[5] is nevertheless an heir of Black liberation theology, a theology that identifies God as a God of the oppressed, one who has a preferential option for the oppressed (namely Black people) and who co-struggles with Black women (and Black people) to bring about their complete social, political, and economic liberation, well-being, and health.[6]

What makes this theology womanist is that it takes it shape from Black women's lived experiences of with the divine, their God talk and their cultural hermeneutic of reading themselves as Black women into biblical scriptures. What also makes the Christian theology many Black women with breast cancer cling to womanist is that it is rooted in a history of Black women's God consciousness and witness of God's presence in their lives under brutal systems of oppression like chattel slavery, segregation, and Jim Crow. Passed down from their foremothers, Black women with breast cancer cling to the faith in God of their foremothers, refashioning it to shape their present circumstances.

Undergirded by their faith in God, the women in this study, like the title of the anthropologist Zora Neale Hurston's womanist novel, are Black women for whom, in breast cancer, *Their Eyes Were Watching God*.[7] These women are looking for God and expecting God to show up in the troubles that breast cancer and intersectional oppressions life brings. And even when they do not always understand God, for them God never fails. God shows up, not just to walk with them through breast cancer, but also to triumph over breast cancer. How God shows up for them becomes clear through their God talk, the way Black women with breast cancer articulate their womanist theology. For them God shows up and God shows out.

God shows up and shows out functioning as a cultural symbol, revealing truths about the ontological, economic, and immanent nature of God. God for some is a liberator, a redeeming force that brings them through and out of breast cancer's troubles. For other Black women with breast cancer, God is a judge, one who calls them to reappraise their lives and makes a way out of no way, giving them access to new ways of living. Black women's faith in God, as part of a womanist theological tradition, is the epistemological lens through which they see, know, and understand breast cancer. As practical theologians, their God talk is how they articulate and theorize what they know.

More than just a way of knowing, Black women's faith in God also functions as the source of their strength. Black women with breast cancer draw strength from believing in God, particularly in the death and resurrection of Jesus. In Jesus Christ, out of his humanity and divinity, Black women with breast cancer find an ally and co-sufferer who understands the troubles Black women face—namely, fears about recurrence and death. By identifying with Jesus's example, Black women write themselves into Jesus's death and resurrection. Jesus overcame death; so can Black women with breast cancer can overcome death. No longer feared, even death no longer has the power to oppress Black women with breast cancer because their theology dictates that death and suffering are not what God intend for them. Jesus rose from the dead, and through their faith, so can Black women with breast cancer. This is the other important aspect of Black women cancer survivors' womanist theology examined in this text. God does not just intervene by reassuring Black women that God is present with them through breast cancer. God shows up to challenge Black women to trouble what troubles them.

As part of their womanist Christian theology, Black women respond to breast cancer by using their pain and allowing it to transform them into change agents.[8] Because God is real in breast cancer, African American cancer survivors respond to breast cancer in culturally distinct ways. Instead of giving up, Black cancer survivors choose to speak up about breast cancer, their faith in God, and what it means to them. They speak up as much to help themselves as they do to help others. Telling their stories is part of what heals them. But Black breast cancer survivors do more than just tell their cancer stories. African American women are also transformed by breast cancer. For these women and those they represent, they become people they never thought possible. Even when breast cancer recurs or is terminal, African American breast cancer survivors remain resolute about God. God is with them in breast cancer, from the diagnosis until death and even after death. This resolute faith in God serves as the core of Black breast cancer survivors' complex hope one that provides psychological comfort to survivors because it is grounded in their Black foremothers' faith in God.[9] Beyond providing emotional support, this complex hope shapes who Black women become as breast cancer survivors and how they operate in the world.

When African American women are transformed by breast cancer into cancer survivors, their actions often turn toward making community for themselves and for others. In these community-making spaces, African American breast cancer survivors emotionally unburden themselves, define themselves, and develop oppositional consciousness in response to breast cancer. All of these efforts are with the intent of achieving health and well-being. As defined by the National Black Women's Health Project,

> ["Health" is] not merely the absence of illness, but the active promotion of emotional, mental and physical wellness of this and future generations. Such wellness is impossible without individual and group empowerment. Such personal and collective empowerment is essential to the redefining and reinterpretation of who Black women are, were and can become.[10]

Part of Black women's unburdening to achieve health and well-being is learning to overcome traps like the Strong Black Woman schema and those set by breast cancer culture, which demand Black women breast cancer survivors' strength be evidenced as silence, piety, dissemblance, and suffering.[11] In response, Black women with breast cancer learn how to holler out so that others recognize their pain and can draw lessons for healing from their experiences with breast cancer.[12] Whether it is through telling their stories or organizing efforts to help others, African American cancer survivors find strength and healing as leaders in their connections and solidarity with others. For them, God is present in the connections they make us leaders.

What African American cancer survivors seem to discover through their interactions with others is that survival serves a greater purpose for them. That greater purpose is to use their survivorship to help others. Black women, in lived response to their womanist theology, become leaders.[13] Even in this, they see God's intervention. God allows them to survive breast cancer so that they can teach others how to survive through tough situations. Nothing in these cancer survivors' experiences is without purpose. This is how they understand God as an economic trinity. God takes all situations—even painful ones—and uses them for a greater purpose. By tapping power, which

Mitchem defines as "a form of cultural creativity to take control of their own lives," Black women use their faith and spirituality to craft their hope.[14] Confident about God's active and supportive presence in their lives, these Black breast cancer survivors fashion their faith into a hope that sustains. It is a theology of complex hope borne out of womanist theology and understood through womanist anthropology that reshapes breast cancer, not as an illness meant for bad, but one meant ultimately for Black women's good. This complex theology of hope is African American breast cancer survivors' theology of health and well-being, a theology that challenges the troubles breast cancer brings.

NOTES

1. Williams, D. (1993). *Sisters in the Wilderness: The Challenge of Womanist God-Talk.* Maryknoll, NY: Orbis Books.
2. Brondo, K. (2010). *Women's Leadership in Anthropology.* Thousand Oaks, CA: SAGE Publications.
3. McClaurin, I. (Ed.). (2002). *Black Feminist Anthropology.* New Brunswick, NJ: Rutgers University Press.
4. Crenshaw, K. (1989). Demarginalizing the Intersection of Race and Sex: A Black Feminist Critique of Antidiscimination Doctrine, Feminist Theory and Antiracist Politics. *University of Chicago Legal Forum*, 139–167; and Collins, P. (2000). *Black Feminist Thought: Knowledge, Consciousness, and the Politics of Empowerment.* New York: Routledge.
5. Grant, J. (1989). *White Women's Christ and Black Women's Jesus: Feminist Christology and Womanist Response.* Atlanta: Scholars Press; and Williams, D. (1993). *Sisters in the Wilderness: The Challenge of Womanist God-Talk.* Maryknoll, NY: Orbis Books.
6. Cone, J. (2003). *God of the Oppressed.* Maryknoll, NY: Orbis Books; Cone, J. (1997). *Black Theology & Black Power.* Maryknoll, NY: Orbis Books; and Cone, J. (2011). *The Cross and the Lynching Tree.* Maryknoll, NY: Orbis Books.
7. Hurston, Z. N. (1975). *Their Eyes Were Watching God.* New York: Doubleday.
8. Lorde, A. (1984). "Eye to Eye: Black Women, Hatred, and Anger." In *Sister Outsider*, 171–172. Trumansburg, NY: Crossing Press; and Townes, E. (Ed.). (1993). "Living in the New Jerusalem: The Rhetoric and Movement of Liberation in the House of Evil." In *A Troubling in my Soul: Womanist Perspectives on Evil & Suffering*, 78–91. Maryknoll, NY: Orbis Books.
9. Ernst, K. (2017). "Terror of Hope: The Integration of Attachment Theory and Womanist Theology." *Pastoral Psychology*, *66*, 201–212.
10. National Black Women's Health Project. (1995). "Definition of Health." *Vital Signs*, *11* (3): 3.
11. Gatison, A. (2015). "The Pink and Black Experience: Lies That Make Us Suffer in Silence and Cost Us Our Lives." *Women's Studies in Communication*, *38*, 135–140.
12. Crawford, A. E. (2002). *Hope in the Holler: A Womanist Theology.* Louisville, KY: Westminister John Knox Press.
13. Smooth, W. (2010). "Intersectionalities of Race and Gender and Leadership." In K. O'Connor (Ed.), *Gender and Women's Leadership: A Reference Handbook*, vol. 1, 31–40. Thousand Oaks: SAGE Publication.
14. Mitchem, S. (2004). *African American Women Tapping Power and Spiritual Wellness.* Cleveland: Pilgrim Press.

Bibliography

Abrams, Jasmine, Morgan Maxwell, Michell Pope, and Faye Belgrave. "Carrying the World with the Grace of a Lady and the Grit of a Warrior: Deepening Our Understanding of the 'Strong Black Woman' Schema." *Psychology of Women Quarterly* 38, no. 4 (2014): 503–518.

Admuyiwa, F., A. Groman, T. O'Connor, C. Ambrosone, N. Watroba, and S. B. Edge. "Impact of Body Mass Index on Clinical Outcomes in Triple Negative Breast Cancer." *Cancer* (2011): 4132–4140.

Amirikia, K., P. Mills, J. Bush, and L. Newman. "Higher Population-Based Incidence Rates of Triple-Negative Breast Cancer among Young African American Women: Implications for Breast Cancer Screening Recommendations." *Cancer* 17, no. 12 (2011): 2747–2753.

American Cancer Society. *Breast Cancer Facts & Figures 2017–2018.* Atlanta: American Cancer Society, 2017.

———. *Cancer Facts & Figures for African Americans 2011–2012.* Atlanta: American Cancer Society, 2011.

———. *Cancer Facts & Figures for African Americans, 2016–2018.* Atlanta: American Cancer Society, 2016.

Armstrong, K., E. Micco, A. Carney, J. Stopfer, and M. Putt. "Racial Differences in the Use of BRCA1/2 Testing among Women with a Family History of Breast or Ovarian Cancer." *JAMA* 293 (2005): 1729–1736.

Augustine. "On the Trinity." In *The Christian Theology Reader*, edited by Alister McGrath. Malden, MA: Wiley-Blackwell, 2011.

Bailey, Zinzi, Nancy Krieger, Madina Agenor, Jasmine Graves, Natalia Linos, and Mary T. Bassett. "Structural Racism and Health Inequities in the USA: Evidence and Interventions." *Lancet* 389 (2017): 1453–1463.

Beauboeuf-Lafonrant, Tamara. *Behind the Mask of the Strong Black Woman: Voice and the Embodiments of a Costly Performance.* Philadelphia: Temple University Press, 2009.

———. "Listening Past the Lies That Make Us Sick: A Voice-Centered Analysis of Strength and Depression among Black Women." *Qualitative Sociology* 31 (2008): 391–406.

Bennis, W., and B. Nanus. *Leaders: Strategies for Taking Charge.* 2nd ed. New York: Harper & Row Publishing, 1997.

Berger, P., and T. Luckman. *The Social Construction of Reality.* Garden City, NY: Anchor, 1966.

Bickell, N. A., J. Neuman, K. Fei, R. Franco, and K. A. Joseph. "Quality of Breast Cancer Care: Perception Versus Practice." *Journal of Clinical Oncology* 30, no. 5 (2012): 1791–1795.

Blaes, A., M. Kreitzer, C. Torkelson, and T. Haddad. "Nonpharmacologic Complementary Therapies in Symptom Management for Breast Cancer Survivors." *Seminars in Oncology* 38 (2011): 394–402.
Brondo, Keri. *Women's Leadership in Anthropology.* Thousand Oaks, CA: SAGE Publications, 2010.
Brown, E. "Womanist Consciousness: Maggie Lena Walker and the Independent Order of Saint Luke." In *Unequal Sisters: A Multicultural Reader in U.S. Women's History*, edited by V. Ruiz and E. DuBois, 268–283. New York: Routledge, 1994.
Brown-Douglass, K. *The Black Christ.* Maryknoll, NY: Orbis Books, 1995.
———. "Womanist Theology: What Is Its Relationship to Black Theology?" In *Black Theology: A Documentary History*, vol. 2, *1980–1992*, edited by James Cone and G. Wilmore, 290–299. Maryknoll, NY: Orbis Books, 1993.
Burns, J. M. *Leadership.* New York: Harper & Row Publishing, 1978.
Carter, Harold. *The Prayer Tradition of Black People.* Valley Forge, PA: Judson Press, 1976.
Caruso, D., J. Mayer, and P. Salovey. "Emotional Intelligence and Emotional Leadership." In *Multiple Intelligences and Leadership*, edited by R. Riggio, S. Murphy, and F. Pirozzolo, 55–74. Mahwah, NJ: Lawrence Erlbaum, 2002.
Charon, Rita. *Narrative Medicine: Honoring the Stories of Illness.* Oxford: Oxford University Press, 2006.
Chen, J., A. Vargas-Bustamante, K. Mortensen, and A. Ortega. "Racial and Ethnic Disparities in Health Care Access and Utilization under the Affordable Care Act." *Medical Care* 54, no. 2 (2016): 140–146.
Citrin, Dennis, Diane Bloom, James Grutsch, Sara Mortensen, and Christopher Lis. "Beliefs and Perceptions of Women with Newly Diagnosed Breast Cancer Who Refused Conventional Treatment in Favor of Alternative Therapies." *The Oncologist* 17 (2012): 607–612.
Collins, Patricia Hill. *Black Feminist Thought.* New York: Routledge, 2000.
———. *Fighting Words: Black Women and the Search for Justice.* Minneapolis: University of Minnesota Press, 1998.
Cone, James. *Black Theology & Black Power.* Maryknoll, NY: Orbis Books, 1997.
———. *God of the Oppressed.* Maryknoll, NY: Orbis Books, 2003.
———. *The Cross and the Lynching Tree.* Maryknoll, NY: Orbis Books, 2011.
Crawford, A. Elaine Brown. *Hope in the Holler: A Womanist Theology.* Louisville, KY: Westminister John Knox Press, 2002.
Crenshaw, Kimberle. "Demarginalizing the Intersection of Race and Sex: A Black Feminist Critique of Antidiscrimination Doctrine, Feminist Theory and Antiracist Politics." *University of Chicago Legal Forum* (1989): 139–167.
Deckman, M. "Women as Leaders in Protestant Denominations." In O'Connor, *Gender and Women's Leadership: A Reference Handbook*, vol. 1, edited by Karen O'Connor, 544–551. Thousand Oaks, CA: SAGE Publishing, 2010.
DeSantis, C. E., S. A. Fedewa, A. Goding Sauer, J. L. Kramer, R. A. Smith, and A. Jamal. "Breast Cancer Statistics, 2015: Convergence of Incidence Rates between Black and White Women." *CA: A Cancer Journal for Clinicians* 66, no.1 (2015): 31–42.
Division of Christian Education of the National Council of Churches of Christ in the U.S.A. *New Revised Standard Version Bible.* New York: HarperCollins Publishers, 1989.
Drew, Elaine, and Nancy Schoenberg. "Deconstructing Fatalism: Ethnographic Perspectives on Women's Decision Making about Cancer Prevention and Treatment." *Medical Anthropology Quarterly* 25, no. 2 (2011): 164–182.
Dunnavant, S. *Celebrating Life: African American Women Speak Out about Breast Cancer.* Dallas: USFI, 1995.
Durkheim, Emile. *The Elementary Forms of the Religious Life.* Translated by Joseph Wardwain. London: George Allen & Unwin, 1976.
Epps, J. C. "On Cancer and Conjuring." In White, *The Black Women's Health Book: Speaking for Ourselves*, 1994, 38–43.
Ernst, Katie. "Terror of Hope: The Integration of Attachment Theory and Womanist Theology." *Pastoral Psychology* 66 (2017): 201–212.
Floyd-Thomas, Stacey, ed. *Deeper Shades of Purple.* New York: NYU Press, 2006.

———. Womanist Ethical Language Handout. April 19, 2017.

Forman, Andrea, and Michael Hall. "Influence of Race/Ethnicity on Genetic Counseling and Testing for Hereditary Breast and Ovarian Cancer." *The Breast Journal* 15, no. s1 (2009): 56–62.

Foucault, Michel. *Discipline & Punish: The Birth of the Prison.* Translated by Alan Sheridan. New York: Random House, 1995.

———. *Power/Knowledge: Selected Interviews and Other Writings, 1972–1977.* Edited by C. Gordon. New York: Pantheon Books, 1980.

Freeman, H. P., and K. C. Chu. "Determinants of Cancer Disparities: Barriers to Cancer Screening, Diagnosis, and Treatment." *Surgical Oncology Clinics of North America* 14 (2005): 655–669.

Gatison, Annette. "The Pink and Black Experience: Lies That Make Us Suffer in Silence and Cost Us Our Lives." *Women's Studies in Communication* 38 (2015): 135–140.

Geertz, Clifford. *Local Knowledge: Further Essays in Interpretive Anthropology.* New York: Basic Books, 1983.

Gerend, Mary, and Manacy Pai. "Social Determinants of Black-White Disparities in Breast Cancer Mortality: A Review." *Cancer Epidemiology, Biomarkers & Prevention* 17, no. 11 (2008): 2913–2923.

Gilkes, C. T. *If It Wasn't for the Women: Black Women's Experience and Womanist Culture in Church and Community.* Maryknoll, NY: Orbis Books, 2001.

———. "Womanist Ways of Seeing." In *Black Theology: A Documentary History*, vol. 2, *1980–1992*, edited by Cone and Wilmore, 1993, 321–324.

Grant, Jacquelyn. *White Women's Christ and Black Women's Jesus: Feminist Christology and Womanist Response.* Atlanta: Scholars Press, 1989.

———. "Women's Experience Revisited: The Challenge of the Darker Sister." In *White Women's Christ and Black Women's Jesus*, 195–230.

Grenz, S. J., and N. L. Erskine. "How Do We Know What to Believe? Revelation and Authority." In *Essentials of Christian Theology*, edited by W. C. Placher, 20–32. Louisville, KY: Westminster, 2003.

Gullatte, M., O. Brawley, A. Kinney, B. Powe, and K. Monney. "Religiosity, Spirituality, and Cancer Fatalism Beliefs on Delay in Breast Cancer Diagnosis in African American Women." *Journal of Religion and Health* 49, no. 1 (2010): 62–72.

Hair, B. Y., S. Hayes, C. K. Tse, A. F. Olshan, and M. B. Bell. "Racial Differences in Physical Activity among Breast Cancer Surviors: Implications for Breast Cancer Care." *Cancer* 120 (2014): 2174–2182.

Halbert, C. H., L. Kessler, A. B. Troxel, J. E. Stopfer, and S. Domcheck. "Effects of Genetic Counseling and Testing for BRCA1 and BRCA2 Mutations in African American Women: A Randomized Trial." *Public Health Genomics* 13 (2010): 440–448.

Hall, W. J., et al. "Implicit Racial/Ethnic Bias among Health Care Professionals and Its Influence on Health Care Outcomes: A Systematic Review." *American Journal of Public Health* 105, no. 12 (2015): e60–76.

Hamilton, J., K. V. Galbraith, N. C. Best, V. Worthy, and A. Moore. "African-American Cancer Survivors' Use of Religious Beliefs to Positively Influence Utilization of Cancer Care." *Journal of Religion & Health* 54 (2015): 1856–1869.

Hamilton, J. B., A. D. Moore, K. A. Johnson, and H. G. Koening. "Reading the Bible for Guidance, Comfort, and Strength during Stressful Life Events." *Nursing Research* 62, no. 3 (2013): 178–184.

Hamilton, J. B., M. Sandelowski, A. D. Moore, M. Agarwal, and H. G. Koenng. "'You Need a Song to Bring You Through': The Use of Religious Songs to Manage Stressful Life Events." *Gerontologist* 53, no. 1 (2013): 26–38.

Hamilton-Mason, J. J. C. Hall, and J. E. Everette. "And Some of Us Are Braver: Stress and Coping among African American Women." *Journal of Human Behavior in the Social Environment* (2009): 463–482.

Harrington, Ellen, Janis Crowther, and Julian Shipherd. "Trauma, Binge Eating, and the 'Strong Black Woman.' *Journal of Counseling and Clinical Psychology* 78, no. 4 (2010): 469–479.

Harris-Lacewell, M. "No Place to Rest: African American Political Attitudes and the Myth of Black Women's Strength." *Women and Politics* 23 (2001): 1–33.

Henneghan, Ashley, and Tracie Harrison. "Complementary and Alternative Medicine Therapies as Symptom Management Strategies for the Late Effects of Breast Cancer Treatment." *Journal of Holistic Nursing* 33, no. 1 (2015): 84–97.

Higginbotham, Evelyn. "The Black Church: A Gender Perspective." In *African American Religion: Interpretive Essays in History and Culture*, edited by T. Fulop and A. Raboteau, 201–225. New York: Routledge, 1997.

———. *Righteous Discontent: The Women's Movement in the Black Church, 1880–1920.* Cambridge, MA: Harvard University Press, 1993.

Hill, S. A. "Cultural Images and the Health of African American Women." *Gender and Society* 23, no. 6 (2009): 733–746.

Hine, Darlene. *Hine Sight: Black Women and the Re-construction of American History.* Bloomington: Indiana University Press, 1994.

hooks, bell. *Feminist Theory: From Margin to Center.* 2nd ed. Cambridge, MA: South End Press, 2000.

Horneber, M., G. Bueschel, G. Dennert, D. Less, E. Ritter, and M. Zwahlen. "How Many Cancer Patients Use Complementary and Alternative Medicine: A Systematic Review and Metaanalysis." *Integrative Cancer Therapies* 11 (2012): 187–203.

Howlader, N., et al. "SEER Cancer Statistics Review, 1975–2012." November 2014. http://seer.cancer.gov/csr/1975_2012/ (accessed July 3, 2017).

Hurston, Z. N. *Their Eyes Were Watching God.* New York: Doubleday, 1975.

Institute of Medicine. *Unequal Treatment: Confronting Racial and Ethnic Disparities in Health Care.* Edited by Brian Smedly, Adrienne Stith, and Alan Nelson. Washington, DC: National Academies Press, 2003.

Irigaray, P., et al. "Lifestyle-Related Factors and Environmental Agents Causing Cancer: An Overview." *Biomedicine & Pharmacotherapy* 61 (2007): 640–658.

Jackson, R., and E. Richardson, eds. *Understanding African American Rhetoric: Classical and Contemporary Innovations.* New York: Routledge, 2003.

Johnson, K. S., K. J. Elbert-Avila, and J. A. Tulsky. "The Influence of Spiritual Beliefs and Practices on the Treatment Preferences of African Americans: A Review of the Literature." *Journal of the American Geriatrics Society* 53 (2005): 711–719.

Jones, Serene. *Feminist Theory and Christian Theology: Cartographies of Grace.* Minneapolis: Fortress Press, 2000.

Kleinman, Arthur. *The Illness Narratives: Suffering, Healing and the Human Condition.* New York: Basic Books, 1988.

Lambe, Camille. "Complementary and Alternative Therapy Use in Breast Cancer: Notable Findings." *Journal of Christian Nursing* 30, no. 4 (2013): 219–225.

Lannin, D., H. Mathews, J. Mitchell, M. Swanson, F. Swanson, and M. Edwards. "Influence of Socioeconomic Status and Cultural Factors on Racial Differences in Late-Stage Presentation of Breast Cancer." *JAMA* 279 (1998): 1801–1807.

Lannin, D. R., H. F. Mathews, J. Mitchell, and M. S. Swanson. "Impacting Cultural Attitudes in African-American Women to Decrease Breast Cancer Mortality." *American Journal of Surgery* 184 (2002): 418–423.

Lee, C. K. *For Freedom's Sake: The Life of Fannie Lou Hamer.* Urbana: University of Illinois Press, 1999.

Lewis, L. "Spiritual Assessment in African-Americans: A Review of Measures of Spirituality Used in Health Research." *Journal of Religion & Health* 47 (2008): 458–475.

Ligibel, J. "Obesity and Breast Cancer." *Oncology* 25 (2011): 994–1000.

Lindbeck, George. *The Nature of Doctrine: Religion and Theology in the Postliberal Age.* Louisville, KY: Westminster John Knox Press, 2009.

Locke, John. *The Second Treatise on Civil Government.* Amherst, MA: Prometheus Books, 1989.

Lorde, Audre. *The Cancer Journals.* Argyle, NY: Spinsters Ink, 1980.

———. "Eye to Eye: Black Women, Hatred, and Anger." In *Sister Outsider*, 171–172. Trumansburg, NY: Crossing Press, 1984.

Lukavsky, R., and J. Sariego. "Insurance Status Effects on Stage of Diagnosis and Surgical Options Used in the Treatment of Breast Cancer." *Southern Medical Journal* 108, no. 5 (2015): 258–261.

Maccartney, S., A. Bishaw, and K. Fontenot. "Poverty Rates for Selected Detailed Race and Hispanic Groups by State and Place: 2007–2011; American Community Survey Briefs." American Community Series Brief/11-17. Economics and Statistics Administration US Department of Commerce. February 2003. http://www.census.gov/prod/2013pubs/acsbr11-17.pdf (accessed May 21, 2018).

Marbury, Herbert. *Pillars of Cloud and Fire: The Politics of Exodus in African American Biblical Interpretation.* New York: New York University Press, 2015.

Mattis, Jacqueline. "African American Women's Definitions of Spirituality and Religiosity." *Journal of Black Psychology* 26 (2000): 101–122.

———. "Religion and Spirituality in the Meaning-Making and Coping Experiences of African American Women: A Qualitative Analysis." *Psychology of Women Quarterly* 26 (2002): 309–321.

McClaurin, I., ed. *Black Feminist Anthropology.* New Brunswick, NJ: Rutgers University Press, 2002.

McGrath, Alister. "The Doctrine of the Trinity." In *Christian Theology: An Introduction*, 234–264. Oxford: Blackwell, 2007.

McKay, N. "Nineteenth-Century Black Women's Spiritual Autobiographies: Religious Faith and Self-Empowerment." In *Interpreting Women's Lives: Feminist Theory and Personal Narrative*, edited by Personal Narratives Group, 139–154. Bloomington: Indiana University Press, 1989.

Meeks, Douglas. "Creation." Lecture presented DIV 2656, Constructive Christian Theology, Nashville, November 1, 2012.

———. "Jesus Christ—Questions." Lecture presented DIV 2656, Constructive Christian Theology, Nashville, October 16, 2012.

———. "Knowing God: Sources and Norms: Scripture, Tradition, Reason and Experience." Lecture presented DIV 2656, Constructive Christian Theology, Nashville, September 2012.

———. "Redemption." Lecture presented DIV 2656, Constructive Christian Theology, Nashville, November 8, 2012.

———. "The Authority and Criticism of Scripture." Lecture presented DIV 2656, Constructive Christian Theology, Nashville, September 2012.

Migliore, D. *Faith Seeking Understanding: An Introduction to Christian Theology.* Grand Rapids, MI: William B. Eerdmans, 2004.

Mitchem, Stephanie. *African American Women Tapping Power and Spiritual Wellness.* Cleveland: Pilgrim Press, 2004.

Moltmann, J. *Theology of Hope: On the Ground and the Implications of Christian Eschatology.* Minneapolis: Fortress Press, 1967.

Moore, Moses. "'Testifying' and 'Testimony': Autobiographcal Narratives and African American Religions." In *Teaching African American Religions*, edited by Carolyn Jones and Theodore Louis Trist, 95–108. Oxford: Oxford University Press, 2005.

Moore, R. J. "African American Women and Breast Cancer: Notes from a Study of Narrative." *Cancer Nursing* (2001): 35–43.

Morgan, P., I. Tyler, and J. Fogel. "Fatalism Revisited." *Seminars in Oncology Nursing* (2008): 237–245.

Mouw, R. J., and T. Peters. "Where Are We Going: Eschatology." In *Essentials of Christian Theology*, edited by W. C. Placher. Louisville, KY: Westminster John Knox Press, 2003.

Moyer, V., and U.S. Preventive Services Task Force. "Risk Assessment, Genetic Counseling, and Genetic Testing for BRCA-Related Cancers in Women: U.S. Preventive Services Task Force Recommendations Statement." *Annals of Internal Medicine* 160, no. 4 (2014): 271–281.

Musgrave, C., C. Allen, and G. Allen. "Spirituality and Health for Women of Color." *American Journal of Public Health* 92 (2002): 557–560.

National Black Women's Health Project. "Definition of Health." *Vital Signs* 11, no. 3 (1995): 3.

Neufeldt, V., and D. Guarlnik, eds. *Webster's New World Dictionary*, 3rd ed. New York: Simon & Schuster, 1998.

Neuhouser, Marian, et al. "Use of Complementary and Alternative Medicine and Breast Cancer Survival in the Health, Eating, Activity and Lifestyle Study." *Breast Cancer Research and Treatment* 160 (2016): 539–546.

Newlin, K., M. Knafl, and G. Melkus. "African-American Spirituality: A Concept Analysis." *Advances in Nursing Science* 25, no. 2 (2002): 57–70.

Newman, Lisa, and Linda Kaljee. "Health Disparities and Triple-Negative Breast Cancer in African American Women: A Review." *JAMA Surgery* (2017): 485–493.

Park, C., and S. Folkman. "Meaning in the Context of Stress and Coping." *Review of General Psychology* 1 (1997): 115–144.

Parks, S. *Fierce Angels: The Strong Black Woman in American Life and Culture.* New York: Random House, 2010.

Parsons, Talcott. *The Social System.* Glencoe, IL: Free Press, 1951.

Peters, Ted. *God—The World's Future: Systematic Theology for the New Era.* 3rd ed. Minneapolis: Augsburg Fortress, 2015.

Pittinsky, T., L. Bacon, and B. Welle. "The Great Women Theory of Leadership? Perils of Positive Streotypes and Precarious Pedestals." In *Women and Leadership: The State of Play and Strategies for Change*, edited by B. Kellerman and D. Rhode, 93–127. San Francisco: Jossey-Bass, 2007.

Porter, J. *Leading Ladies: Transformative Biblical Images of Women's Leadership.* Philadelphia: Innisfree Press, 2000.

Powe, B., E. Daniels, and R. Finnie. "Comparing Perceptions of Cancer Fatalism among African American Patients and Their Providers." *Journal of the Academy of Nursing Practice* (2005): 318–324.

Robnett, Belinda. *How Long? How Long? African American Women and the Struggle for Civil Rights.* New York: Oxford University Press, 1997.

———. "Women Leaders in the Civil Rights Movement." In O'Connor, *Gender and Women's Leadership: A Reference Handbook*, vol. 1, 2010, 196–203.

Rogers, Eugene. "Where the Spirit Rests: Matter and Narrative." In *After the Spirit: A Constructive Pneumatology from Resources Outside the Western World.* Grand Rapids, MI: William B. Eerdmans Publishing, 2005.

Rosser-Mims, Dionne. "Black Feminism: An Epistemological Framework for Exploring How Race and Gender Impact Black Women's Leadership Development." *Advancing Women in Leadership Journal* 30, no. 15 (2010): 1–10.

Rousseau, Jean-Jacques. *Basic Political Writings.* Translated by D. Cress. Indianapolis: Hackett, 1987.

———. *The Government of Poland.* Translated by W. Kendall. Indianapolis: Hackett, 1985.

Scott, J. *Weapons of the Weak: Everyday Forms of Peasant Resistance.* New Haven, CT: Yale University Press, 1985.

Shaw, Stephanie. *What a Woman Ought to Be and to Do: Black Professional Women Workers during the Jim Crow Era.* Chicago: University of Chicago Press, 1996.

Sheppard, Vanessa, Darren Mays, Thomas LaVeist, and Kenneth Tercyak. "Medical Mistrust and Self-Efficacy Influence Black Women's Level of Engagement in BRCA1/2 Genetic Counseling and Testing." *Journal of the National Medical Association* 105, no. 1 (2013): 17–22.

Siegel, D. J., and M. Hartzell. *Parenting from the Inside Out: How a Deeper Self-Understanding Can Help You Raise Children Who Thrive.* New York: Penguin Group, 2003.

Siegel, Rebecca, Kimberly Miller, and Ahmedin Jemal. "Cancer Statistics, 2018." *CA: A Cancer Journal for Clinicians* 68 (2018): 7–30.

Skinner, C. S., C. L. Arfken, and R. K. Sykes. "Knowledge, Perceptions, and Mammography Stage of Adoption among Older Urban Women." *American Journal of Preventive Medicine* 14 (1998): 54–63.

Smooth, Wendy. "Intersectionalities of Race and Gender and Leadership." In O'Connor, *Gender and Women's Leadership: A Reference Handbook*, vol. 1, 2010, 31–40.

Snyder, C. R. "Hope Theory: Rainbows in the Mind." *Psychological Inquiry* 13, no. 4 (2002): 249–275.

Stolley, M., L. Sharp, A. Wells, N. Simon, and L. Schiffer. "Health Behaviors and Breast Cancer: Experiences of Urban African American Women." *Health Education & Behavior* 33 (2006): 604–624.

Su, S., et al. "The Quality of Invasive Breast Cancer Care for Low Reimbursement Rate Patients: A Retrospective Study." *PLoS ONE* 12, no. 9 (2017): 1–13.

Sulik, G. A. *Pink Ribbon Blues: How Breast Cancer Culture Undermines Women's Health.* New York: Oxford University Press, 2010.

Tate, Johnettea. "The Role of Spiritualty in the Breast Cancer Experiences of African American Women." *Journal of Holistic Nursing* 29, no. 4 (2011): 249–255.

Taylor, E. J. "Transformation of Tragedy among Women Surviving Breast Cancer." *Oncology Nursing Forum* 27, no. 5 (2000): 781–788.

Taylor, T. R., C. D. Williams, and K. H. Makambi. "Racial Discrimination and Breast Cancer Incidence in US Black Women: The Black Women's Health Study." *American Journal of Epidemiology* 166 (2007): 46–54.

Thompson, C. L., C. Owusu, N. L. Nock, L. Li, and N. A. Berger. "Race, Age, and Obesity Disparities in Adult Physical Activity Levels in Breast Cancer Patients and Controls." *Frontiers in Public Health* 2 (2014): 150.

Townes, Emilie. "Living in the New Jerusalem: The Rhetoric and Movement of Liberation in the House of Evil." In *A Troubling in My Soul: Womanist Perspectives on Evil & Suffering*, 78–91. Maryknoll, NY: Orbis Books, 1993.

Tronto, Joan. *Moral Boundaries: A Political Argument for an Ethic of Care.* New York: Routledge, 1993.

Ucok, O. "The Fashioned Survivor: Institutionalized Representations of Women with Breast Cancer." *Communication and Medicine* 4, no. 1 (2007): 67–78.

Vetter, Lisa. "Overview: Feminist Theories of Leadership." In O'Connor, *Gender and Women's Leadership: A Reference Handbook*, vol. 1, 2010, 3–10.

Walker, Alice. "In Search of Our Mothers' Gardens." In Cone and Wilmore, *Black Theology: A Documentary History*, vol. 1, *1960–1979*, 1993, 339–346.

Ward, B. W., T. C. Clarke, G. J. Freeman, and J. S. Schiller. "Early Release of Selected Estimates Based on Data from the 2014 National Health Interview Survey." *Centers for Disease Control and Prevention.* June 2015. https://www.cdc.gov/nchs/data/nhis/earlyrelease/earlyrelease201506.pdf (accessed May 21, 2018).

Weems, Renita. *Just a Sister Away: Understanding the Timeless Connection Between Women of Today and Women in the Bible.* New York: Warner, 1989.

White, E., ed. *The Black Women's Health Book: Speaking for Ourselves.* Seattle: Seal Press, 1990.

Williams, Charles, and Hilda Williams. "Mutual Aid Societies and Economic Development: Survival Efforts." In *African Amercians in the South: Issues of Race, Class and Gender*, edited by Hans Baer and Yvonne Jones. Athens: University of Georgia Press, 1992.

Williams, Delores. *Sisters in the Wilderness: The Challenge of Womanist God-Talk.* Maryknoll, NY: Orbis Books, 1993.

Wood, Frances. "'Take My Yoke upon You': The Role of the Church in the Oppression of African-American Women." In Townes, *A Troubling in My Soul: Womanist Perspectives On Evil & Suffering*, 2003, 37–47.

Woods-Giscombe, Cheryl. "Superwoman Schema: African American Women's Views on Stress, Strength and Health." *Qualitative Health Research* 20, no. 5 (2010): 668–683.

Yedjou, Clement, et al. "Assessing the Racial and Ethnic Disparities in Breast Cancer Mortality in the United States." *International Journal of Environmental Research and Public Health* 14, no. 486 (2017): 1–14.

Young, Marion. *Inclusion and Democracy.* New York: Oxford University Press, 2000.

Zhang, Y., L. Franzini, W. Chan, H. Xu, and X. L. Du. "Effects on Health Insurance on Tumor Stage, Treatment, and Survival in Large Cohorts of Patients with Breast and Colorectal Cancer." *Journal of Health Care for the Poor and Underserved* 26, no. 4 (2015): 1336–1358.

Index

Anita, 136, 147n55
anthropology : anthropologist's roles, ix, 4; ethnographic research, 150; examining cultural theology, 4; immersion into Black women's lives, ix, x; praxis of anthropological theologian, xi; study of illness narratives, 45; study methodology, 4
Atkins, Karla, 76, 83n16; meaning of breast cancer for, 76–77; support for another cancer survivor, 77–79

Bernice, 131, 140
Black Church: recognizing Black women as leaders, 95, 96, 97; support for cancer survivors, x, 31–32, 60, 66, 67, 102; testifying in, 44, 52
Black Feminist/Womanist Anthropology: consequence for scientific inquiry, 5, 150; study methodology, 4, 152
Black women : cancer survivorship leaders, 88, 153; change agents, 127, 152; inside expert theologians, 126; self-defined standpoint, 88, 99; social marginalization of, 75; stereotyped as fatalists, 73; victim to change agent, 74–75, 81, 82, 87
Black women's breast cancer disparity : BRCA 1/ BRCA 2 genetic testing and discrimination, 101; culture as risk for, 8, 73–74; diminishing life as a result of, 79, 82; healthcare provider perceptions as risk for, 9; incidence as, 5–6; mortality as, 6, 82, 125; poverty as risk for, 7–8; racial discrimination as risk for, 8–9, 9; survivorship stigma as, 50, 114, 115, 116, 119; triple-negative breast cancer as, 6–7
Black women's cancer support seeking : breast cancer culture's impact on, 57; cultural patterning of, 58–71; desire for racial concordance, 63–64; fashioned survivor impact on, 57; family and friends' roles in, 57–58, 102, 103–104; mutual aid in, 59–61, 66–67, 71; silence in, 55–56; Strong Black Woman schema impacts on, 55–57, 58; survivor examples of, 102–104, 105–106; resistance towards white cancer networks, 107
Black women's cancer testimonies : alleviate emotional distress, 48, 113; bolster faith, 45; cultural productions, 43; God's role in, 43, 44; illness narratives, 45; structure of, 43, 45; testifying as component of, 33, 43–44, 47–48, 48–49, 52; voicing how God functions, 43; web of significance, 43; wellness strategy, 44, 44–45, 48–49. *See also* cancer testimonies
Black women researchers : advocates for Black women, ix; responsibilities to

cancer survivors, ix
Black women's spirituality and religiosity : faith in God as component of, 73–75, 79, 80, 82–83, 125, 151–152; God talk as part of, 46–47, 104, 105–106, 106; response to discrimination, 10; religiosity definition, 11; religious involvement as resource for, 11–12; spirituality definition, 10; spirituality of survival, 60, 68, 69, 99; tapping power of, 153. *See also* Black women's theology; Black women's cancer testimonies; Christian theology
Black women's theology : Black women's troubles as part of, 5, 10, 12, 126, 128, 136–137, 143, 150; cultural epistemology of, 2; cultural theology as, 4, 5, 12, 73–75, 128; constructive theology as, 19, 41; God as cultural symbol for, 1; God as metaphor in, 21–22; God in community with Black women, 133; God talk as part of, 3, 33, 35, 36, 39–40, 126–128; God's response to troubles in, 3, 10, 11, 75, 126, 128, 129, 134–135, 136–137, 139, 145, 151–152; God who stands for life, 75; Holy Spirit as part of, 2; identification with crucified and resurrected Jesus as part of, 74, 82, 87, 129; identification with triune God, 1–3; Jesus as Black woman in, 3; Jesus as part of, 2; Jesus' identification with oppressed in, 2–3; ontological awareness as part of, 127, 132–133; practical theology, 3, 126, 128; resources for, 20, 33, 35–36, 39, 95, 127–128, 128, 130–132; ways of knowing God, 1. *See also* Christian theology; God (constructions of); Black women's spirituality and religiosity
breast cancer: late-stage disease and faith, 75–76; life-changing experience of, 87; like religious conversion experience, 87; oppositional consciousness about, 60; recurrence, 75, 77–78; stigma as a result of, 49, 114; viewed as tragedy, 112, 115
breast cancer survivorship: leadership resulting from, 87–88; new life perspective in, 87; thriving roles as epistemology of, 120–121

cancer testimonies : benefits for diagnosis and treatment, 45; reasons for giving, 49–50, 51–52; reasons for not giving, 49–50, 50; rewards of giving, 50–51; risks associated with, 50; wellness strategy, 44, 45, 48–49, 52. *See also* Black women's cancer testimonies
Cheryl, 135, 137, 140, 147n58
Christian Theology : cultural system, 19; God's roles in, 1, 149; resources for, 20, 127–128, 128, 130–132; talking about God part of, 21, 22. *See also* Black women's theology; God (constructions of)
clergy : support for cancer survivors, x–xi, 31, 32, 60, 65, 67–68
complex hope : Black women's, 129–130; definition of, 129; different from eschatological hope, 129, 139, 141; different from optimistic hope, 129; holler as expression of, 130; recognition of living dead in relation to, 144; theology of, 141–142. *See also* hope
Constance, 125, 143, 145n1
cultural theology of well-being, 126–127. *See also* Black women's theology; Black women's cancer testimonies; cancer testimonies; hope; complex hope

death (including dying): Black women facing, 3, 75, 88; lack of denial about, 75; support for loved one's, 78–79; refusal to fear, 80–81
dissemblance (masking): impact on Black women's health, 56, 58, 62, 70–71; culture of, 57, 69; masking true feelings as, 57, 58, 62, 63, 67, 67–68, 69–71; resistance to oppression as, 69–70; response to anger towards God as, 63, 67–68

Eunice, 143–144, 148n100

fatalism : barrier to cancer treatment, 73–74; connected to faith in God, 73, 80; definition of, 73; refusal to fear as response to, 81; response to cancer disparities, 82

God (constructions of) : co-sufferer with Black women, 79, 80, 82, 98, 125–126, 126, 129, 133, 138, 151; economic Trinity for, 135, 136, 138, 153; healer, 32, 40, 79; judge, 21–28, 40, 98; liberator, 21–22, 29–40, 40, 98, 109, 134, 135, 136, 137–138. *See also* Black women's theology; Christian theology; God (constructions of)

Glover, Hattie, 26, 41n10; breast cancer as God's judgment, 26–27, 28; constructive theology, 25, 26–28; God as lenient judge, 26, 27, 28

Harris, Carlice, 49, 53n11, 83n17; reasons for testifying, 49, 50, 51–52; reasons for not testifying, 49–50, 50; refusal to fear death, 80–81; rewards of testifying, 50–51; testifying as risky endeavor, 50

health-care providers : advocates for Black women, ix; Black health care providers' responsibilities to survivors, ix; experiences with, 34, 35, 37, 38, 45, 64–65, 78; hidden transcripts not shared with, 76, 82; patient narratives' benefits for, 45

hidden transcripts : distinct from public transcripts, 76; function as counter-narratives, 76; God in relation to, 76, 79, 80. *See also* resistance

Holmes, Hilda, 112, 124n77; breast cancer as tragedy, 112, 115; cancer testimony, 113, 114, 117; experience with cousin's death, 113, 117; seeking healer leadership of, 112–120; self-perception as leader, 114, 118–119; self-perception as weak, 112, 114, 115, 116, 119

hope: Black women's views of God as, 125, 129; cancer survivor testimonies as, 45; response to breast cancer disparities, 125; theological resource, 125; visionary pragmatism as, 129. *See also* complex hope

Hudson, Virginia, 23, 41n9; breast cancer as God's judgment, 24, 25; breast cancer as God's rehabilitation of life, 25; constructive theology, 23–25; reappraisal of God, 25

Knox, Felicia, 101, 123n64; BRAC 1/ BRAC 2 gene carrier, 101; decision to forego adjuvant therapy, 101; supporting seeking, 102, 103–104, 105–106; survivorship and leadership, 103; spiritualty and leadership, 104–105; use of complementary and alternative medicine, 102; views of social support for survivors, 105, 106–107; weaving leadership of, 106–109

leadership : Black women's, 88, 93–94, 95, 96–97, 98; Black feminist/womanist theory and, 93–96, 97; Black women's authority in, 88; Black women's response to oppression, 93; bridge leaders, 95; ethic of care as, 91, 98, 120; etymology of, 88; female biblical archetypes of, 89, 95, 97, 110–111, 119; feminist theory and, 88, 92–96; intersectionality in relation to, 93–94; ideas about women and, 89–96; leading ladies, 88, 89; outsider within as epistemology for, 94; seeking healer as example of, 100, 110–120; self-awareness as part of, 88; transformative leadership, 97–98, 98–99, 100; transformative model of, 97–98, 99; weaver as example of, 100–110; womanist ethics of, 98, 99, 107, 108; womanist theology and, 95

Marlo, 134, 139, 146n43

mutual aid : African Americans' historical use of, 58–59; context for survivors' use of, 59–61; cultural functions of, 59–60, 61; definition of, 60; resource for oppositional consciousness, 60; support for emotional transparency, 65–66, 71; survivors' uses of, 64, 66, 66–68, 69, 71; processing emotions through, 65–68, 71. *See also* Black women's support seeking

nommo (generative power of spoken word), 56, 109, 144

pain : breast cancer as source of, 82; definition of, 74; detachment as response to, 46, 70; different from suffering, 74; fuel for struggle, 74; God who co-struggles with, 82; internalization of, 46, 47, 56; suppressed emotions, 46–47. *See also* suffering

resistance : counter-narratives as, 75–76; persistence in living as, 79–80, 82–83; refusal to fear death as, 80–81; reliance on God as, 76, 79; response to breast cancer, 74–75, 79–80; response to dying as, 79–80; silence about God as, 73

Renee, 143, 145, 148n99

Roxanne, 141, 147n87

Sandra, 140, 147n77

Scott, Melba, 29, 41n11; constructive theology, 29–33; God's liberation through prayer, 30–31, 32; importance of testimony, 30, 31, 33

social support : provided as divine mission, 103, 104, 105, 105–106. *See also* Black women's cancer support seeking; Black women's cancer testimonies; mutual aid

Sparks, Tracy, 62, 72n22; anger at God, 67–68, 71; learning to dissemble, 69–70, 71; masking true feelings (dissemblance), 62–63, 67, 69–71; reappraisal of God, 67–69

spirituality of survival, 60, 68, 69, 99; feelings about God part of, 69; Felicia Knox and, 108–109; leadership roles as reflection of, 97–99, 108. *See also* Black women's spirituality and religiosity

Strong Black Woman schema : controlling image of Black women, 9, 55, 56, 91; God in relation to, 134; impact on Black women's health, 56, 58, 62, 67; internalization of pain, 56; masking feelings, 46, 55–56, 69, 70; overcoming, 153; problem for Black women, 9; resistance to oppression, 69–70; silence as component of, 55–56, 56, 57, 68. *See also* dissemblance (masking)

suffering : breast cancer as source of, 82; different from pain, 74; part of cultural theology, 74; resistance to, 74; sin as, 74, 82; transformed into wholeness, 87. *See also* pain

Wanda, 145, 148n105

womanist theology : Black women's response to troubles as, 151; consequence for scientific inquiry, 5, 12; study methodology, 4, 149

Young, Krystal, 33, 42n14, 45, 53n10; anger with God, 36, 39, 46, 47; betrayal by God, 47; constructive theology, 33, 34–40; scripture as theological resource, 33, 35–36, 39; cancer testimony, 46–47; reasons for testifying, 47–48, 48; testifying as wellness strategy for, 48–49

About the Author

Dr. Elizabeth A. Williams received her PhD and MA degrees in applied anthropology with an emphasis in medical anthropology from the University of Kentucky. She received her BA degree, also in anthropology, from the University of Illinois, Urbana-Champaign. Dr. Williams further holds graduate reading certificates in behavioral science and women's studies from the University of Kentucky. After receiving her doctorate, Dr. Williams served on the faculty in the Department of Anthropology and Geography at Georgia State University, as the inaugural Director of Disparity Elimination for the Tennessee Department of Health, and as a senior-level administrator with the Vanderbilt-Ingram Cancer Center. Dr. Williams is an associate professor in the Department of Public Health, Health Administration, and Health Sciences at Tennessee State University. She has completed fellowships with the Kellogg Foundation Emerging Leader in Public Health Program; Cal Turner Program for Moral Leadership; Vanderbilt University Divinity School; the African American Mental Health Research Scientist Consortium, sponsored by the National Institute of Mental Health and the American Evaluation Association. Presently a Branson Fellow (2008–present), Rev. Dr. Williams is pursuing a MDiv degree from Vanderbilt University Divinity School and is a licensed pastor in the United Methodist Church, currently serving as associate pastor at Clark Memorial United Methodist Church in Nashville, Tennessee.

www.ingramcontent.com/pod-product-compliance
Lightning Source LLC
Chambersburg PA
CBHW031414220926
51612CB00004B/11